MIND DIET COOKBOOK FOR SENIORS

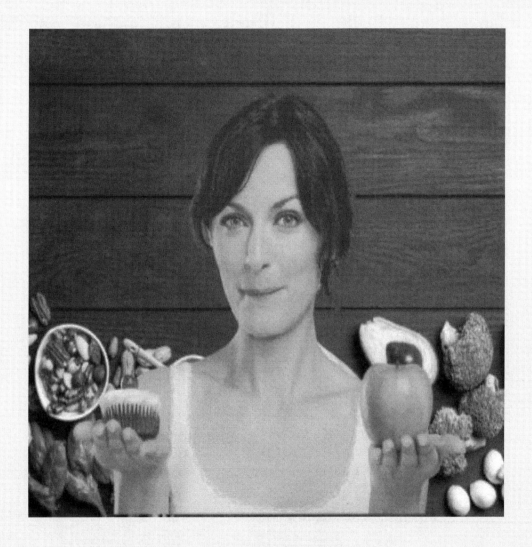

The Ultimate Guide On Making Delicious and Easy-to-make Recipes To Help You Improve Your Memory and Reduce Your Risk Of Alzheimer's Disease

Anne J. Henderson

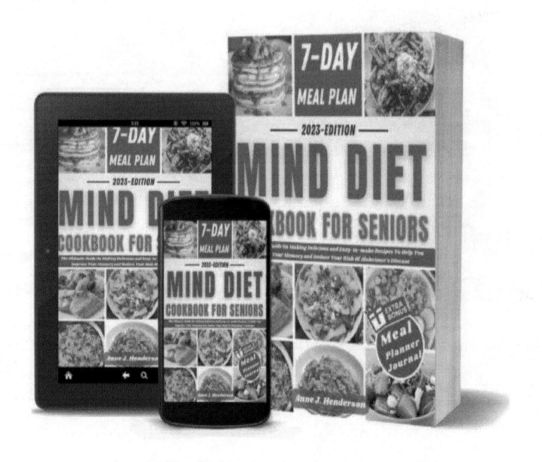

Table Of Contents

INTRODUCTION

Caroline was a 65-year-old woman who had been diagnosed with Alzheimer's disease a few years ago. She had always been a devoted chef, and she loved spending time in the kitchen. But as her sickness worsened, she found it more and more difficult to recall recipes, and she would frequently forget what she was doing in the midst of cooking.

One day, Caroline's daughter, Sarah, stumbled upon a cookbook that was made exclusively for persons with Alzheimer's disease. The cookbook was loaded with basic, easy-to-follow recipes, and it also featured memory-boosting activities that could be done while cooking.

Sarah decided to give the cookbook a try, and she was shocked at how much it benefited her mother. Caroline was able to recall the recipes more quickly, and she also felt that the memory exercises helped to enhance her general cognitive performance.

As Caroline continued to use the cookbook, she witnessed a tremendous improvement in her memory. She was able to cook more independently, and she even began to experiment with new dishes. She also started to engage in more activities outside of the kitchen, and her general quality of life improved dramatically.

Note:

Caroline's experience is a testimonial to the potential of cognitive stimulation in the treatment of Alzheimer's disease. The correct cookbook may be a great tool for persons with Alzheimer's, and it can assist to enhance their memory, their cognitive function, and their quality of life.

So What Are You Waiting For?

Continue Reading This Book To Find More About Improving Your Brain Function.

Welcome To This Book "Mind Diet Cookbook For Seniors"

About The Book

The MIND diet is a dietary pattern that has been found to lessen the risk of Alzheimer's disease and dementia. This cookbook is meant to help seniors follow the MIND diet by presenting them with tasty and easy-to-make dishes.

This cookbook is a fantastic resource for anybody who wishes to enhance their brain health. It is particularly useful for elderly, who are at an elevated risk of Alzheimer's disease and dementia. The dishes are tasty and simple to create, and they can be customized to match your personal dietary demands.

A Letter From The "Author"

I hope that this cookbook will enable you to enhance your brain health and lower your chances of Alzheimer's disease and dementia. I think that everyone has the right to live a long and healthy life, and I want to do my bit to help make that happen.

I feel that this book has the potential to benefit a lot of individuals. I hope that you will find it beneficial and that you will utilize it to better your own brain health.

CHAPTER ONE

Understanding MIND Diet

The MIND diet is a mix of the Mediterranean diet and the DASH diet, and it is supposed to help prevent Alzheimer's disease and other kinds of dementia. The MIND diet stresses eating lots of fruits, vegetables, whole grains, nuts, legumes, and seafood, while reducing saturated fat, red meat, and processed foods.

The MIND diet is based on the premise that specific foods may help protect the brain from harm and boost cognitive performance. The foods that are highlighted on the MIND diet are rich in antioxidants, vitamins, minerals, and other nutrients that are vital for brain function.

Some of the particular items that are advised on the MIND diet include:

- **Fruits:** Berries, apples, pears, oranges, bananas, and grapes
- **veggies:** Leafy greens, cruciferous veggies (like broccoli and Brussels sprouts), tomatoes, onions, and garlic
- **Whole grains:** Whole-wheat bread, brown rice, quinoa, and oats
- **Nuts:** Almonds, walnuts, peanuts, and pistachios
- **Beans:** Black beans, kidney beans, lentils, and chickpeas
- **Fish:** Salmon, tuna, trout, and mackerel

The MIND diet also allows for a modest amount of red meat and dairy, but it excludes processed meals, sugary beverages, and bad fats.

The MIND diet is a healthy and nutritious way to eat, and it may also help protect your brain from harm. If you are interested in attempting the MIND diet, there are numerous materials accessible online and in libraries.

The Science Behind the MIND Diet

The MIND diet was devised expressly to safeguard brain function, and early research shows that it may be successful in doing so.

The MIND diet focuses on foods that are high in antioxidants, vitamins, and minerals that are regarded to be advantageous for brain function. These foods include:

- Green leafy veggies
- Other veggies
- Nuts Berries Beans
- Whole grains
- Seafood Poultry
- Olive oil
- Wine

The MIND diet also avoids harmful foods that might lead to inflammation and oxidative stress, which are both known to be risk factors for Alzheimer's disease and other kinds of dementia. These foods include:

- Red meat
- Butter with stick margarine
- Cheese Pastries and desserts
- Fried/fast food

There has been a number of research studies that have studied the relationship between the MIND diet and cognitive deterioration. One research, published in the journal Alzheimer's & Dementia, indicated that persons who followed the MIND diet had a 53% reduced risk of Alzheimer's disease than those who did not follow the diet. Another research, published in the journal Neurology, indicated that persons who followed the MIND diet had a slower rate of cognitive deterioration than those who did not follow the diet.

The MIND diet is a pretty straightforward diet to follow, and it is based on items that are already part of many people's diets.

Here are some of the proposed processes via which the MIND diet may preserve brain health:

1. Antioxidants: The MIND diet is rich in antioxidants, which may help protect cells from harm caused by free radicals. Free radicals are unstable chemicals that may harm cells, and they are suspected to have a role in the development of Alzheimer's disease and other kinds of dementia.

2. Polyphenols: The MIND diet also includes high quantities of polyphenols, which are plant components that have antioxidant and anti-inflammatory effects. Polyphenols have been found to increase cognitive performance and protect against neurodegenerative disorders.

3. Omega-3 fatty acids: The MIND diet contains oily fish, which are an excellent source of omega-3 fatty acids. Omega-3 fatty acids have been demonstrated to boost cognitive performance and protect against Alzheimer's disease.

4. Flavonoids: The MIND diet also contains berries, which are an excellent source of flavonoids. Flavonoids have been demonstrated to boost cognitive performance and protect against Alzheimer's disease.

Overall, the MIND diet is a good nutritional strategy for safeguarding brain function. More study is required to validate the long-term advantages of the MIND diet, but it is a safe and simple method to improve your diet and possibly lower your risk of Alzheimer's disease and other kinds of dementia.

The Benefits Of The MIND Diet To Seniors

Here are some of the advantages of the MIND diet:

1. Reduces the risk of Alzheimer's disease and dementia. Studies have revealed that persons who follow the MIND diet are at a decreased risk of getting Alzheimer's disease and dementia. In one research, participants who followed the MIND diet had a 53% reduced risk of Alzheimer's disease than those who did not follow the diet.

2. Improves cognitive function. The MIND diet may also assist enhance cognitive performance in elderly persons. In one research, those who followed the MIND diet for five years exhibited gains in their memory, attention, and executive function.

3. Protects against heart disease and stroke. The MIND diet is also healthy for your heart and circulatory system. It may help lessen your risk of heart disease, stroke, and other cardiovascular disorders.

4. Promotes weight loss. The MIND diet is a nutritious and balanced diet that may help you lose weight or maintain a healthy weight.

5. May help prevent cancer. Some studies have shown that the MIND diet may possibly help prevent cancer.

The MIND diet is a simple and effective strategy to boost your brain function and general wellbeing. If you are seeking a strategy to minimize your risk of Alzheimer's disease, dementia, heart disease, stroke, and cancer, the MIND diet is an excellent alternative.

How To Follow The MIND Diet

The MIND diet is a brain-healthy eating regimen that combines the DASH and Mediterranean diets. It has been demonstrated to lessen the risk of Alzheimer's disease and cognitive impairment.

Here are some recommendations on how to follow the MIND diet:

1. Eat lots of fruits and veggies. The MIND diet emphasizes consuming a variety of fruits and vegetables, particularly green leafy vegetables, berries, and beans. Aim to consume at least 5 servings of fruits and vegetables every day.

2. Choose whole grains over processed grains. Whole grains are a rich source of fiber, which may assist to enhance heart health and cognitive function. Choose whole-wheat bread, brown rice, quinoa, and other whole grains whenever feasible.

3. Eat fish frequently. Fish is an excellent source of omega-3 fatty acids, which have been found to protect the brain from harm. Aim to consume fish at least 1-2 times a week.

4. Limit saturated and harmful fats. The MIND diet advocates minimizing saturated fat and harmful fats, such as those found in butter, margarine, cheese, and pastries. Instead, pick healthy fats, such as those found in olive oil, avocados, and almonds.

5. Drink lots of fluids. Water, tea, and coffee are all healthy alternatives for fluids. Avoid sugary liquids, such as soda and juice.

6. Limit alcohol consumption. The MIND diet advocates limiting alcohol consumption to one glass per day for women and two glasses per day for males.

Here are some things to avoid on the MIND diet:

- Butter
- Margarine
- Cheese
- Red meat
- Fried food
- Pastries
- Sweets

The MIND diet is a reasonably straightforward diet to follow. It is adaptable enough to fit into most lifestyles and may be tailored to your own tastes. If you are searching for a strategy to boost your brain health, the MIND diet is a wonderful choice to explore.

CHAPTER TWO

7 DAYS meal plan

7 Day Mind Diet Meal Plan

Day 1

Breakfast

Oatmeal with berries and nuts

Lunch

Salad with grilled chicken or fish, chickpeas, and olive oil dressing

Dinner

Salmon with roasted vegetables

Day 2

Breakfast

Whole-wheat toast with avocado and eggs

Lunch

Lentil soup with a side salad

Dinner

Chicken stir-fry with brown rice

Day 3

Breakfast

Yogurt with berries and granola

Lunch

Tuna salad sandwich on whole-wheat bread

Dinner

Vegetarian chili with cornbread

Day 4

Breakfast

Smoothie with berries, spinach, and yogurt

Lunch

Leftover vegetarian chili

Dinner

Roasted chicken with potatoes and green beans

Day 5

Breakfast

Whole-wheat pancakes with fruit

Lunch

Salad with beans and quinoa

Dinner

Salmon with roasted sweet potatoes

Day 6

Breakfast

Eggs with whole-wheat toast and avocado

Lunch

Leftover salmon with roasted sweet potatoes

Dinner

Lentil soup with a side salad

Day 7

Breakfast

Oatmeal with berries and nuts

Lunch

Salad with grilled chicken or fish, chickpeas, and olive oil dressing

Dinner

Veggie burger on a whole-wheat bun with sweet potato fries

This is just a sample meal plan, and you can adjust it to fit your own preferences and dietary needs. Be sure to include a variety of fruits, vegetables, whole grains, and healthy fats in your diet. You can also include a glass of wine with dinner, but limit it to one glass per day.

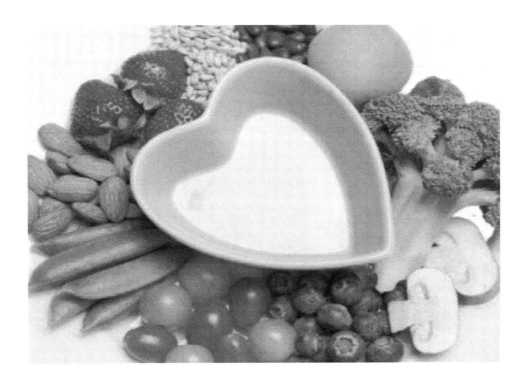

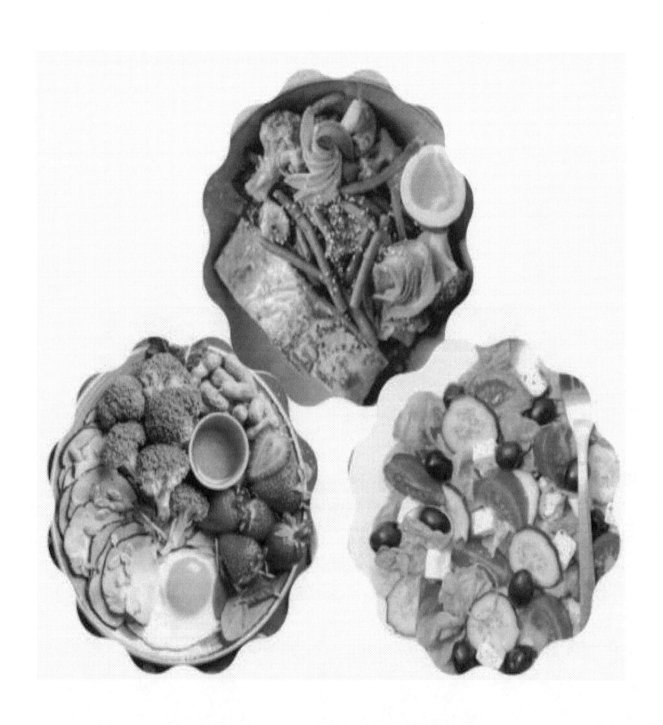

Breakfast, Lunch, & Dinner

CHAPTER THREE

Healthy And Delicious Mind Diet Recipes For Seniors

Energizing Breakfast Recipes

1. Eggs Benedict with whole-wheat English muffins

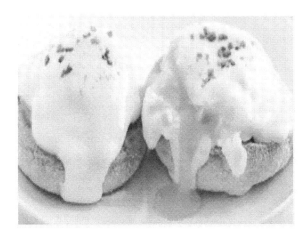

Eggs Benedict is a famous brunch meal that is created with poached eggs, Canadian bacon, and hollandaise sauce, all served on an English muffin. This recipe includes whole-wheat English muffins to make it a healthier alternative.

Preparation Time: 15 minutes
Cooking Time: 10 minutes
Total Time: 25 minutes

Ingredients:

- 2 whole-wheat English muffins, split and toasted
- 4 pieces Canadian bacon, cooked
- 4 poached eggs Hollandaise sauce (recipe below)

Instructions:

- To create the hollandaise sauce, melt 1 tablespoon butter in a small saucepan over low heat.
- Whisk in 2 egg yolks and 1 tablespoon lemon juice.
- Gradually whisk in 1 cup of boiling water, 1 teaspoon salt, and 1/4 teaspoon black pepper.
- Cook, whisking continually, until the sauce is thick and creamy.
- To construct the Eggs Benedict, lay a toasted English muffin on each dish.
- Top each muffin with a piece of Canadian bacon, a poached egg, and a liberal quantity of hollandaise sauce.

Nutritional information:

Serve size: 1 serve

- Calories: 728
- Carbohydrates: 48 grams
- Fat: 43 grams
- Protein: 32 grams
- Fiber: 4 grams

Tips

- To poach eggs, bring a big saucepan of water to a simmer.
- Crack each egg into a small basin.
- Gently put the eggs into the hot water.
- Cook for 3-4 minutes, or until the whites are set and the yolks are still runny.
- Use a slotted spoon to take the eggs from the water and drain on paper towels.
- To create hollandaise sauce ahead of time, mix the ingredients together and then cover and chill.
- Reheat the sauce slowly over low heat before serving.

2. Hash browns with black beans and salsa

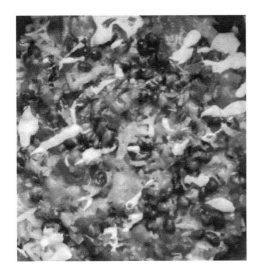

This dish is a wonderful and quick way to start your day. It's created with hash browns, black beans, salsa, and cheese, and it's excellent for a quick and tasty breakfast or brunch.

Preparation Time: 10 minutes

Cooking Time: 15 minutes

Total Time: 25 minutes

Ingredients:

- 1 pound hash browns, thawed if frozen
- 1/2 cup black beans, washed and drained
- 1/4 cup salsa
- 1/4 cup shredded cheddar cheese
- Salt and pepper to taste

Instructions:

- Heat a large skillet over medium heat.
- Add the hash browns and heat, turning periodically, until golden brown and crispy.

- Stir in the black beans, salsa, and cheese.
- Season with salt and pepper to taste.
- Cook for a further 2-3 minutes, or until the cheese is melted and bubbling.
- Serve immediately.

Nutrition:

Serving size: 4

- Calories: 400
- Carbohydrates: 40 grams
- Fat: 15 grams
- Protein: 15 grams
- Fiber: 5 grams

Tips

- For extra crispy hash browns, soak the potatoes in cold water for 30 minutes before cooking.
- If you don't have salsa, you may substitute spicy sauce or your favorite taco sauce.
- Garnish with your favorite toppings, such as sour cream, avocado, or cilantro.

3. Breakfast burrito with eggs, beans, and cheese

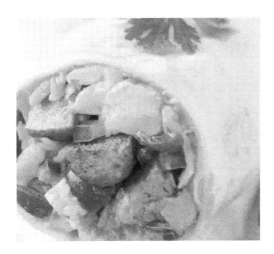

This is a simple and tasty breakfast burrito dish that is excellent for a quick and easy supper. It is created with eggs, beans, cheese, and your favorite toppings. The burritos may be cooked ahead of time and frozen, making them a wonderful alternative for hectic mornings.

Preparation Time: 10 minutes
Cooking Time: 10 minutes
Total Time: 20 minutes

Ingredients:

- 8 big eggs
- 1/4 teaspoon salt
- 1/8 teaspoon black pepper
- 1 tablespoon olive oil
- 1 (15-ounce) can black beans, washed and drained
- 1/4 cup shredded cheddar cheese
- 4 big flour tortillas
- Your favorite toppings, such as salsa, sour cream, guacamole, or avocado

Instructions:

- In a large bowl, mix together the eggs, salt, and pepper.
- Heat the olive oil in a large pan over medium heat. Add the eggs and heat, stirring periodically, until cooked through.
- Stir in the black beans and cheese.
- Warm the tortillas according to the package recommendations.
- To construct the burritos, distribute a layer of the egg mixture down the middle of each tortilla. Top with your favorite toppings.
- Fold the burritos in half and roll them securely.
- Serve immediately or wrap securely in plastic wrap or foil and refrigerate or freeze for later.

Nutritional information:

Serving size: 1 tortilla

- Calories: 450
- Carbohydrates: 45 grams
- Fat: 20 grams
- Protein: 20 grams
- Fiber: 10 grams

Tips

- For a crispier tortilla, fry it in a skillet over medium heat until the outside is golden brown.
- To make ahead, construct the burritos and then cover them firmly in plastic wrap or foil. Refrigerate or freeze for up to 3 days. To reheat, defrost the burritos in the refrigerator overnight or in the microwave for a few minutes. Then, cook them in a pan over medium heat until heated through.
- Get creative with your toppings! Some additional fantastic possibilities are chopped veggies, bacon, sausage, or sour cream.

4. Oatmeal with peanut butter and banana

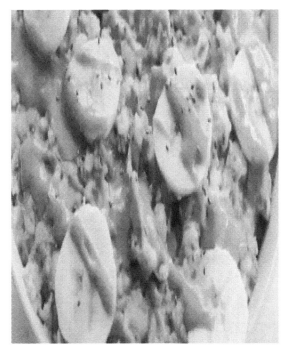

Oatmeal with peanut butter and banana is a tasty and nutritious breakfast choice. It is a rich source of complex carbs, protein, and fiber. The peanut butter lends a creamy richness, while the banana contributes sweetness and moisture. This dish is simple to create and may be tweaked to your desire.

Preparation Time: 5 minutes
Cooking Time: 5 minutes
Total Time: 10 minutes

Ingredients:

- 1 cup old-fashioned oats
- 1 cup milk
- 1/2 cup water
- 1 banana, mashed
- 2 tbsp peanut butter

- 1/2 teaspoon ground cinnamon
- Pinch of salt

Instructions:

- In a medium saucepan, mix the oats, milk, water, banana, peanut butter, cinnamon, and salt.
- Bring the mixture to a boil over medium heat, stirring frequently.
- Reduce the heat to low and simmer for 5 minutes, stirring periodically.
- Serve immediately or let cool and enjoy later.

Nutritional information:

Serving size: 1 cup

- Calories: 375
- Carbohydrates: 55 grams
- Fat: 15 grams
- Protein: 10 grams
- Fiber: 5 grams

Tips

- For a fuller taste, use almond milk or coconut milk instead of ordinary milk.
- Add various toppings, such as chopped nuts, seeds, or fruit, to personalize the taste of your porridge.
- This dish may be prepared ahead of time and kept in the refrigerator for up to 3 days.

5. Whole-wheat cereal with fruit and milk

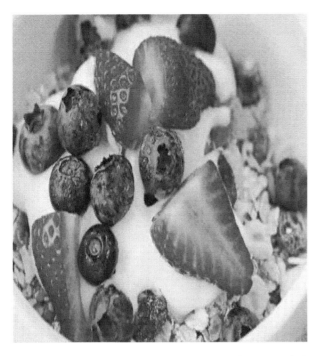

This is a quick and nutritious breakfast meal that is excellent for a hectic morning. It is prepared using whole-wheat cereal, fresh berries, and milk. You may alter the sweetness to your preference by adding more or less honey. This meal is also an excellent source of fiber, protein, and vitamins.

Preparation Time: 5 minutes

Cooking Time: 0 minutes

Total Time: 5 minutes

Ingredients:

- 1 cup whole-wheat cereal
- 1 cup milk
- 1/2 cup fresh berries (such as blueberries, raspberries, or strawberries)
- 1 tablespoon honey (optional)

Instructions:

- In a bowl, mix the cereal, milk, and berries.

- Stir to mix.
- If desired, add the honey.
- Serve immediately.

Nutritional facts per serving:

Serving size: 1 cup

- Calories: 250
- Carbohydrates: 40 grams
- Fat: 5 grams
- Protein: 10 grams
- Fiber: 5 grams

Tips

- You may use whatever sort of whole-wheat cereal you want.
- If you don't have fresh berries, you may substitute frozen berries.
- You may alter the sweetness of the cereal to your desire by adding more or less honey.
- This meal is also an excellent source of fiber, protein, and vitamins.

6. Avocado toast with smoked salmon

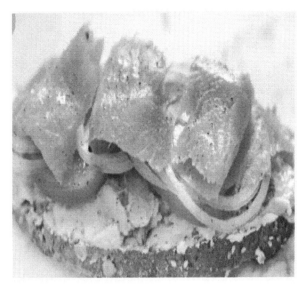

Avocado toast with smoked salmon is a tasty and healthful breakfast or snack. It is fast and simple to cook, and it is filled with nutrients. The avocado delivers healthful fats, fiber, and vitamins, while the smoked salmon is a fantastic source of protein and omega-3 fatty acids.

Preparation Time: 5 minutes
Cooking Time: 0 minutes
Total Time: 5 minutes

Ingredients:

- 2 pieces of bread
- 1/2 avocado, mashed
- 2 ounces smoked salmon
- 1/4 cucumber, thinly sliced
- 1 tablespoon microgreens
- 1/4 teaspoon salt
- 1/8 teaspoon black pepper

Instructions:

- Toast the bread.

- Spread the mashed avocado on the bread.
- Top with the smoked salmon, cucumber, microgreens, salt, and pepper.
- Serve immediately.

Nutritional information:

Serve size: 1 serve

- Calories: 270
- Carbohydrates: 20 grams
- Fat: 15 grams
- Protein: 10 grams
- Fiber: 5 grams

Tips

- For a more tart taste, add a squeeze of lemon juice to the avocado.
- If you don't have microgreens, you may substitute chopped fresh herbs, such as dill or parsley.
- You may also add additional toppings to your avocado toast, such as eggs, bacon, or cheese.

7. Banana bread with walnuts

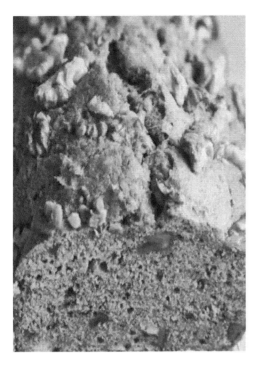

Banana bread is a popular fast bread that is simple to prepare and always a crowd-pleaser. This recipe is for a moist and fragrant banana bread with walnuts, which provides a great crunch and nutty taste.

Preparation Time: 15 minutes
Cooking Time: 50-60 minutes
Total Time: 1 hour

Ingredients:

- 3 ripe bananas, mashed
- ⅓ cup unsalted butter, softened
- ¾ cup sugar
- 1 egg
- 1 teaspoon vanilla extract
- 1 teaspoon baking soda
- ¼ teaspoon salt
- 1 ½ cups all-purpose flour

- ½ cup chopped walnuts

Instructions:

- Preheat the oven to 350 degrees F (175 degrees C). Grease and flour a 9x5 inch loaf pan.
- In a large bowl, mix together the butter and sugar until light and fluffy. Beat in the egg and vanilla extract.
- In a separate dish, mix together the flour, baking soda, and salt. Gradually add to the wet components, mixing until just mixed. Stir in the walnuts.
- Pour batter into the prepared loaf pan and bake for 50-60 minutes, or until a toothpick inserted into the middle comes out clean.
- Let bread sit in the pan for 10 minutes before transferring to a wire rack to cool fully.

Nutrition:

Serving size: 1 slice (1/12 of bread)

Calories: 220

Carbohydrates: 34 grams

Fat: 11 grams

Protein: 4 grams

Fiber: 3 grams

Tips

- For a moist banana bread, use extremely ripe bananas.
- If you don't have walnuts, you may substitute other nuts, such as pecans or almonds.
- To create a chocolate banana bread, add 1/2 cup of chocolate chips to the dough.
- This recipe may be easily doubled to produce a bigger loaf.

8. Yogurt bowl with granola and fruit

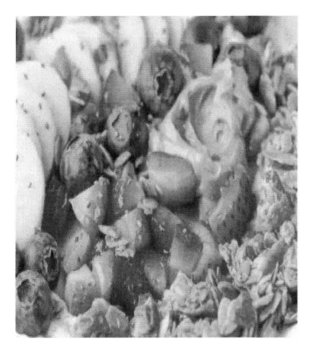

Yogurt bowls are a tasty and nutritious breakfast option that is simple to create. They are created with yogurt, granola, and fresh fruit, and may be personalized to your desire. This recipe is for a simple yogurt bowl, but you may put in additional things like almonds, seeds, honey, or maple syrup.

Preparation Time: 5 minutes

Cooking Time: 0 minutes

Total Time: 5 minutes

Ingredients:

- 1 cup plain yogurt
- 1/2 cup granola
- 1 cup fresh fruit, such as berries, bananas, or peaches
- 1-2 teaspoons honey or maple syrup (optional)

Instructions:

- In a bowl, mix the yogurt, granola, and fruit.
- Drizzle with honey or maple syrup, if preferred.
- Serve immediately.

Nutritional information:

Serving size: 1 dish

- Calories: 350-400
- Carbohydrates: 40-50 grams
- Fat: 10-15 grams
- Protein: 15-20 grams
- Fiber: 5-10 grams

Tips

- Use your favorite kind of yogurt. Greek yogurt is a wonderful option since it is strong in protein.
- Choose a choice of fruits to add to your yogurt dish. This will help you receive a range of nutrients.
- If you are hoping for a sweeter yogurt dish, add a little honey or maple syrup.
- You may also add additional items to your yogurt dish, such as almonds, seeds, or granola.

9. Waffles with strawberries and whipped cream

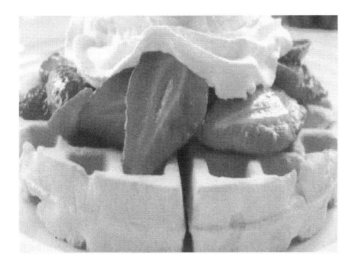

Waffles with strawberries and whipped cream is a popular breakfast or brunch meal that is both tasty and simple to create. The waffles are light and fluffy, the strawberries are sweet and tangy, and the whipped cream is thick and creamy. This dish is excellent for a special occasion or a leisurely weekend morning.

Preparation Time: 15 minutes

Cooking Time: 15 minutes

Total Time: 30 minutes

Ingredients:

- 1 3/4 cups all-purpose flour
- 2 tablespoons baking powder
- 1 teaspoon baking soda
- 1 teaspoon cinnamon
- 1 tablespoon sugar
- 1/4 teaspoon salt
- 2 egg yolks
- 1 3/4 cups milk

- 1/2 cup vegetable oil
- 2 teaspoons vanilla extract
- 2 egg whites
- 1 pound strawberries, sliced
- 2 tablespoons sugar
- 2 cups whipped cream

Instructions:

- In a large basin, mix together the flour, baking powder, baking soda, cinnamon, sugar, and salt.
- In a separate dish, mix together the egg yolks, milk, oil, and vanilla extract.
- Fold the wet ingredients into the dry ingredients until just mixed.
- In a clean dish, whip the egg whites until firm peaks form.
- Fold the egg whites into the batter until barely incorporated.
- Preheat your waffle iron according to the manufacturer's directions.
- Pour 1/4 cup of batter onto the waffle iron and cook until golden brown, according to the manufacturer's recommendations.
- Repeat steps 7 and 8 with the remaining batter.
- In a small dish, mix the strawberries and sugar.
- Serve the waffles with the strawberries and whipped cream.

Nutrition:

Serving size: 4 waffles

- Calories: 450
- Carbohydrates: 55 grams
- Fat: 15 grams
- Protein: 10 grams
- Fiber: 5 grams

Tips

- For extra crispy waffles, preheat your waffle iron in a 250 degree F oven for 5 minutes before cooking.
- If you don't have a waffle iron, you may cook the batter in a big pan over medium heat.
- To make the strawberries especially sweet, you may add a spoonful of honey or maple syrup to the bowl with the strawberries.
- You may also add additional toppings to your waffles, such as blueberries, bananas, or chocolate chips.

10. Pancakes with blueberries and almonds

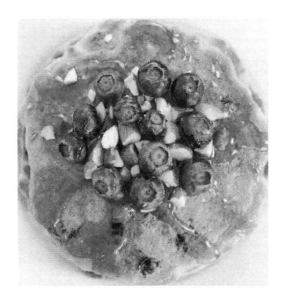

These airy pancakes are baked with fresh blueberries and walnuts, and they're sure to become a family favorite. They're easy to create and just need a few basic ingredients. Serve them with your favorite toppings, like maple syrup, butter, or fresh fruit.

Preparation Time: 10 minutes

Cooking Time: 15 minutes

Total Time: 25 minutes

Ingredients:

- 1 1/2 cups all-purpose flour
- 2 tablespoons baking powder
- 1 teaspoon baking soda
- 1 teaspoon sugar
- 1/2 teaspoon salt 1 cup buttermilk
- 1 big egg, beaten
- 2 teaspoons melted butter
- 1/2 cup frozen blueberries
- 1/3 cup chopped walnuts

Instructions:

In a large bowl, mix together the flour, baking powder, baking soda, sugar, and salt.

In a separate dish, mix together the buttermilk, egg, and melted butter.

Pour the wet ingredients into the dry ingredients and whisk until barely mixed. Do not overmix.

Stir in the blueberries and walnuts.

Heat a big skillet or griddle over medium heat. Grease the pan with butter or cooking spray.

Pour 1/4 cup of batter into the heated pan for each pancake. Cook for 2-3 minutes each side, or until golden brown.

Repeat steps 5-6 with the remaining batter.

Serve immediately with your preferred toppings.

Nutrition:

Serving Size: Makes 12 pancakes

- Calories: 270
- Carbohydrates: 36 grams
- Fat: 10 grams

- Protein: 7 grams
- Fiber: 3 grams

Tips

- For fluffier pancakes, let the batter rest for 5 minutes before frying.
- If you don't have buttermilk, you may create your own by adding 1 tablespoon of lemon juice or vinegar to 1 cup of milk and letting it settle for 5 minutes.
- To keep the blueberries from sinking to the bottom of the pancakes, mix them with a little flour before adding them to the batter.
- Serve the pancakes with your favorite toppings, such as maple syrup, butter, fresh fruit, or whipped cream

11. Whole-wheat bread with avocado and poached eggs

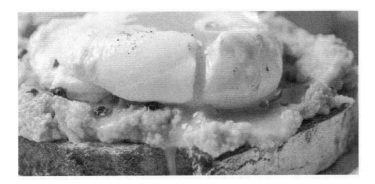

Avocado toast with poached eggs is a tasty and nutritious morning choice. It is rich with nutrients, including healthy fats, fiber, and protein. The avocado provides smoothness and richness, while the poached eggs give a burst of protein. This dish is simple to create and may be tweaked to your desire.

Preparation Time: 5 minutes

Cooking Time: 5 minutes

Total Time: 10 minutes

Ingredients:

- 2 slices whole-wheat bread
- 1/2 avocado, mashed
- 2 big eggs
- 1 tablespoon white vinegar
- Salt and pepper to taste

Instructions:

- Toast the bread.
- While the bread is toasting, cook the eggs. To achieve this, bring a small pot of water to a simmer. Add the vinegar and spin the water to form a vortex. Crack one egg into a small basin, then carefully slide the egg into the water. Repeat with the second egg. Cook the eggs for 3-5 minutes, or until the whites are set and the yolks are still runny.
- Remove the eggs from the water with a slotted spoon and drain on paper towels.
- Spread the mashed avocado on the toasted bread.
- Top with the poached eggs and season with salt and pepper to suit.

Nutrition:

Serving size: 2 slices

- Calories: 350
- Carbohydrates: 25 grams
- Fat: 20 grams
- Protein: 15 grams
- Fiber: 5 grams

12. Omelet with feta cheese and avocado

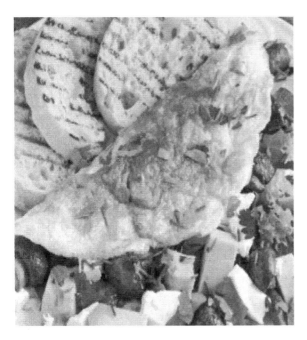

This is a simple and tasty omelet dish that is excellent for breakfast, brunch, or a light meal. The creamy avocado and salty feta cheese make a terrific mix, and the entire meal is ready in only a few minutes.

Preparation Time: 5 minutes

Cooking Time: 5 minutes

Total Time: 10 minutes

Ingredients:

- 2 big eggs
- 1/4 teaspoon salt
- 1/8 teaspoon black pepper
- 1 tablespoon olive oil
- 1/2 avocado, diced
- 1/4 cup feta cheese, crumbled

Instructions:

- In a small bowl, mix together the eggs, salt, and pepper.
- Heat the olive oil in a small nonstick pan over medium heat.
- Pour the egg mixture into the skillet and cook, stirring regularly, until the eggs are set but still wet, approximately 2 minutes.
- Top with the avocado and feta cheese.
- Fold the omelet in half and cook for another minute, or until the cheese is melted.
- Serve immediately.

Nutrition:

Serving size: 1 omelet

- Calories: 270
- Carbohydrates: 10 grams
- Fat: 18 grams
- Protein: 15 grams
- Fiber: 4 grams

Tips

- For a deeper taste, use a mixture of olive oil and butter in the skillet.
- If you don't have feta cheese, you may substitute another sort of salty cheese, such as goat cheese or Parmesan cheese.
- Add some chopped fresh herbs, such as basil or dill, to the omelet for an added blast of flavor.
- Serve the omelet with a side of fruit or bread for a full breakfast.

13. Scrambled eggs with spinach and tomatoes

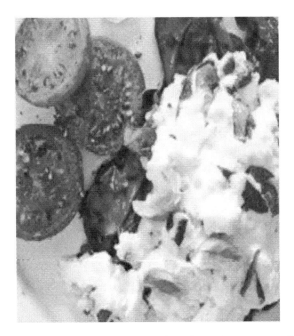

Scrambled eggs with spinach and tomatoes is a quick and simple breakfast or brunch meal that is filled with nutrition. The eggs give protein, the spinach delivers vitamins and minerals, and the tomatoes bring taste and acidity. This recipe is easy to follow and may be tweaked to your desire.

Preparation Time: 5 minutes

Cooking Time: 5 minutes

Total Time: 10 minutes

Ingredients:

- 2 tablespoons olive oil
- 1 cup baby spinach, cleaned and sliced
- 1/2 cup grape tomatoes, halved
- 2 big eggs
- 1 tablespoon water
- Salt and pepper to taste

Instructions:

- Heat the olive oil in a large non-stick skillet over medium heat.
- Add the spinach and tomatoes to the pan and heat until the spinach has wilted, approximately 2 minutes.
- In a small bowl, mix together the eggs and water.
- Pour the eggs into the pan with the spinach and tomatoes and heat, turning regularly, until the eggs are done to your preference.
- Season with salt and pepper to taste.

Nutrition:

Serving Size: 2 servings

- Calories: 250
- Carbohydrates: 15 grams
- Fat: 15 grams
- Protein: 15 grams
- Fiber: 5 grams

Tips

- For a fuller taste, use whole eggs instead of egg whites.
- If you want your eggs more runny, cook them for a shorter length of time.
- Add your favorite toppings, like cheese, bacon, or avocado.

14. Greek yogurt parfait with fruit and almonds

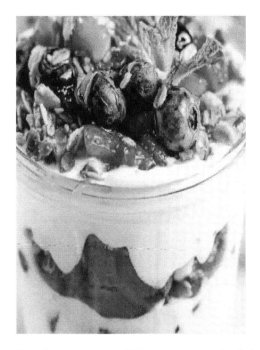

Greek yogurt parfaits are a wonderful and healthful breakfast or snack alternative. They are rich with protein, fiber, and other minerals, and they may be personalized to your desire. This recipe contains plain Greek yogurt, granola, fruit, and almonds, but you may add additional ingredients as desired.

Preparation Time: 5 minutes

Cooking Time: 0 minutes

Total Time: 5 minutes

Ingredients:

- 1 cup plain Greek yogurt
- 1/2 cup granola
- 1/2 cup fresh fruit, such as berries, peaches, or bananas
- 1/4 cup chopped nuts, such as almonds, walnuts, or pecans

Instructions:

- In a glass or dish, layer the yogurt, granola, fruit, and nuts.
- Repeat layering until the parfait is filled.
- Enjoy!

Nutrition:

Serving Size: 1

- Calories: 350
- Carbohydrates: 40 grams
- Fat: 15 grams
- Protein: 15 grams
- Fiber: 5 grams

Tips

- For a sweeter parfait, add a drizzle of honey or maple syrup.
- You may use whatever sort of fruit you want in this recipe.
- If you prefer a nut-free parfait, just eliminate the nuts.
- This recipe may be easily doubled or tripled to produce extra parfaits.

15. Overnight oats with berries

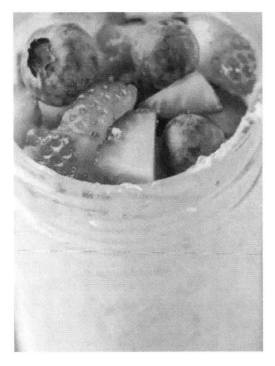

Overnight oats are a quick and simple breakfast that can be cooked ahead of time and eaten on the run. They are a healthy and nutritious meal that is filled with fiber and protein. This recipe for overnight oats with berries is a tasty and simple way to start your day.

Preparation Time: 5 minutes

Cooking Time: None

Total Time: 5 minutes

Ingredients:

- 1/2 cup rolled oats
- 1 cup milk (any variety)
- 1/2 cup Greek yogurt
- 1/2 cup berries (any sort)
- 1 tablespoon chia seeds (optional)
- 1 teaspoon honey (optional)

Instructions:

- In a jar or dish, mix the oats, milk, yogurt, berries, chia seeds, and honey (if using).
- Stir to mix.
- Cover and refrigerate overnight.
- In the morning, stir and enjoy!

Nutrition:

Serving size: 1 jar or bowl

- Calories: 350
- Carbohydrates: 50 grams
- Fat: 10 grams
- Protein: 15 grams
- Fiber: 5 grams

Tips

- You may use any sort of milk in this recipe.
- If you don't have chia seeds, you may skip them or substitute another kind of seed, such as flaxseed or hemp seed.
- You may add additional items to your overnight oats, such as nuts, seeds, or spices.
- Enjoy your overnight oats cold or warm.

1. Black Bean and Sweet Potato Quesadillas

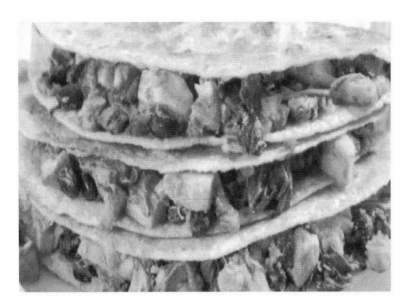

These Black Bean and Sweet Potato Quesadillas are a tasty and simple way to get your daily dose of veggies. They are created with roasted sweet potatoes, black beans, cheese, and your preferred seasonings. Quesadillas are a terrific supper at any time of day, and they are also a great way to use up leftover ingredients.

Preparation Time: 15 minutes

Cooking Time: 20 minutes

Total Time: 35 minutes

Ingredients:

- 1 big sweet potato, peeled and chopped
- 1 tablespoon chili powder
- 1 teaspoon cumin
- 1/2 teaspoon smoked paprika
- 1/4 teaspoon salt

- 1/4 teaspoon black pepper
- 1 (15-ounce) can black beans, drained and rinsed
- 1 cup shredded cheddar cheese
- 6 (8-inch) flour tortillas

Instructions:

- Preheat the oven to 400 degrees F (200 degrees C).
- Toss sweet potato with chili powder, cumin, smoked paprika, salt, and pepper.
- Spread sweet potato mixture evenly on a baking sheet.
- Bake in a preheated oven for 20-25 minutes, or until sweet potatoes are soft and slightly browned.
- While sweet potatoes are baking, heat a large pan over medium heat.
- Place a tortilla in the griddle and top with black beans, cheese, and roasted sweet potatoes.
- Cook for 2-3 minutes each side, or until the cheese is melted and the tortilla is golden brown.
- Repeat with remaining tortillas.
- Serve immediately.

Nutrition:

Serving size: 2 quesadillas

- Calories: 350
- Carbohydrates: 40 grams
- Fat: 15 grams
- Protein: 15 grams
- Fiber: 10 grams

Tips

- For a hotter quesadilla, add a sprinkle of cayenne pepper to the sweet potato mixture.
- Use your preferred sort of cheese in this recipe. I prefer to use cheddar, but you could also use Monterey Jack, pepper jack, or even a Mexican cheese combination.
- Serve these quesadillas with your favorite toppings, such as sour cream, guacamole, salsa, or pico de gallo.
- Leftover quesadillas may be kept in the refrigerator for up to 3 days. To reheat, just microwave them until cooked through.

2. Roasted Vegetable Hummus Wraps

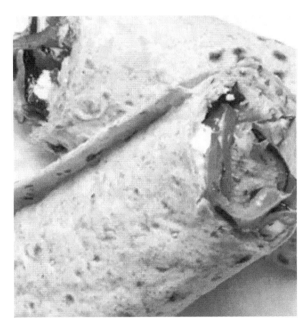

Roasted Vegetable Hummus Wraps are a tasty and nutritious food choice that is excellent for lunch or supper. They are created with roasted veggies, hummus, and your favorite leafy greens. The wraps are simple to construct and may be adjusted to your desire.

Preparation Time: 15 minutes

Cooking Time: 20 minutes

Total Time: 35 minutes

Ingredients:

- 1 tablespoon olive oil
- 1 red bell pepper, sliced
- 1 yellow bell pepper, sliced
- 1/2 red onion, sliced
- 1 zucchini, sliced
- 1 (15-ounce) can chickpeas, washed and drained
- 1/4 cup tahini
- 3 tablespoons lemon juice
- 1 clove garlic, minced
- 1/2 teaspoon salt
- 1/4 teaspoon black pepper
- 4 whole-wheat tortillas
- Your favorite leafy greens, such as spinach or arugula

Instructions:

- Preheat the oven to 400 degrees F (200 degrees C).
- Toss the bell peppers, onion, and zucchini with the olive oil.
- Spread the veggies on a baking sheet and roast for 20 minutes, or until soft and slightly browned.
- While the veggies are roasting, mix the chickpeas, tahini, lemon juice, garlic, salt, and pepper in a food processor.
- Process until smooth, scraping down the sides as required.
- Spread hummus on the tortillas.
- Top with roasted veggies and lush leaves.
- Roll up the wraps and enjoy.

Nutritions:

Serving Size: 1 wrap

- Calories: 350
- Carbohydrates: 40 grams
- Fat: 15 grams
- Protein: 10 grams
- Fiber: 6 grams

Tips

- For a hotter wrap, add a sprinkle of cayenne pepper to the hummus.
- For a more delicious wrap, roast the veggies with your preferred herbs and spices.
- Serve the wraps with a side of your favorite dipping sauce, such as tzatziki or hummus.

3. Greek Yogurt Chicken Salad Pitas

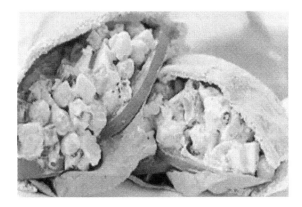

Greek Yogurt Chicken Salad Pitas are a healthy and tasty lunch or supper alternative. They are created with basic ingredients, including Greek yogurt, chicken, veggies, and herbs. The yogurt dressing offers a creamy and savory touch, while the veggies bring freshness and crunch. These pitas are simple to prepare and may be tweaked to your desire.

Preparation Time: 10 minutes

Cooking Time: 0 minutes

Total Time: 10 minutes

Ingredients:

- ¾ cup plain Greek yogurt
- 2 teaspoons lemon juice
- 1 clove garlic, minced
- ¼ teaspoon salt
- ¼ teaspoon black pepper
- 1 teaspoon dill
- 1 cup cucumber, chopped
- 1 bunch green onion, chopped
- 2 cups cooked chicken, shredded or diced
- 2 big whole wheat pitas, split in half

Instructions:

- In a large bowl, mix together the Greek yogurt, lemon juice, garlic, salt, pepper, and dill.
- Stir in the cucumber and green onion.
- Fold in the chicken until thoroughly mixed.
- Divide the chicken salad between the pita halves and serve.

Nutrition:

Serving size: 1 pita half

- Calories: 270
- Carbohydrates: 25 grams
- Fat: 10 grams

- Protein: 25 grams
- Fiber: 5 grams

Tips

- For a lower-calorie alternative, try light Greek yogurt.
- Add more veggies, such as tomatoes, red onion, or celery.
- For a hotter salad, add a sprinkle of cayenne pepper or red pepper flakes.
- Serve with a side of fruit or veggies for a full supper.

4. Chicken and Broccoli Stir-Fry

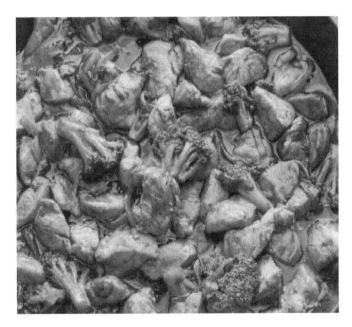

Chicken and broccoli stir-fry is a popular Chinese meal that is fast and simple to cook. It is a nutritious and tasty dish that is excellent for a midweek supper.

Preparation Time: 15 minutes

Cooking Time: 10 minutes

Total Time: 25 minutes

Ingredients:

- 1 pound boneless, skinless chicken breasts, cut into 1-inch pieces
- 2 tablespoons cornstarch
- 1 tablespoon soy sauce
- 1 teaspoon sesame oil
- 1/2 teaspoon black pepper
- 1 tablespoon vegetable oil
- 1 head broccoli, cut into florets
- 1 onion, chopped
- 1 clove garlic, minced
- 1/4 cup chicken broth
- 1 tablespoon soy sauce
- 1 teaspoon brown sugar
- 1/4 teaspoon sesame oil

Instructions:

- In a medium bowl, mix the chicken, cornstarch, soy sauce, sesame oil, and black pepper. Toss to coat.
- Heat the vegetable oil in a large pan or wok over medium-high heat. Add the chicken and heat, moving periodically, until browned and cooked through, approximately 5 minutes.
- Add the broccoli and onion to the skillet and cook, turning periodically, until the broccoli is bright green and tender, approximately 3 minutes.
- In a small bowl, mix together the chicken broth, soy sauce, brown sugar, and sesame oil. Add to the skillet and bring to a boil. Reduce heat to low and simmer for 1 minute, or until the sauce has thickened.
- Serve immediately over rice.

Nutrition:

Serving size: 4

- Calories: 450
- Carbohydrates: 30 grams
- Fat: 15 grams
- Protein: 30 grams
- Fiber: 5 grams

Tips

- You may use any sort of broccoli for this dish. If you want your broccoli softer, you may blanch it in boiling water for 2-3 minutes before adding it to the pan.
- If you don't have chicken broth, you may substitute water or veggie broth.
- You may add additional veggies to this stir-fry, such as carrots, mushrooms, or bell peppers.
- Serve this stir-fry over rice, quinoa, or noodles.

5. Avocado Tuna Salad Sandwiches

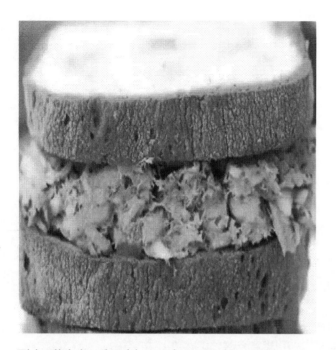

This dish is a healthy and tasty take on the conventional tuna salad sandwich. The avocado offers a creamy richness and a dose of healthful fats, while the celery and red onion add a hint of crispness. This salad is excellent for a fast and simple lunch or supper, and it can be easily adjusted to your desire.

Preparation Time: 10 minutes
Cooking Time: 0 minutes
Total Time: 10 minutes

Ingredients:

- 1 (12-ounce) can albacore tuna, drained and flakes
- 1/2 ripe avocado, mashed
- 1/2 cup celery, chopped
- 1/4 cup red onion, chopped
- 1 tablespoon lemon juice
- 1 teaspoon Dijon mustard

- 1/2 teaspoon salt
- 1/4 teaspoon black pepper
- 4 slices whole wheat bread

Instructions:

- In a medium bowl, add the tuna, avocado, celery, red onion, lemon juice, mustard, salt, and pepper. Mix thoroughly.
- Spread the tuna salad on the bread pieces.
- Serve immediately, or keep in the refrigerator for later.

Nutrition:

Serving size: 1 sandwich

- Calories: 350
- Carbohydrates: 20 grams
- Fat: 20 grams
- Protein: 20 grams
- Fiber: 5 grams

Tips

- For a more acidic taste, add 1 tablespoon of dill pickle relish.
- For a hotter taste, add 1/2 teaspoon of cayenne pepper.
- To prepare the sandwiches ahead of time, assemble them without the bread and keep them in the refrigerator for up to 24 hours. When you're ready to dine, just cover the bread with mayonnaise and top with the tuna salad.

6. Lentil Soup with Spinach and Feta

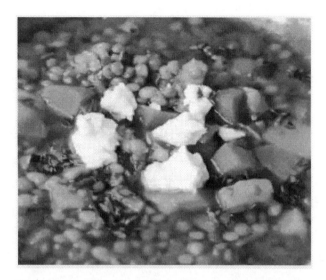

This rich and savory lentil soup is a terrific way to warm yourself on a chilly day. The lentils cook fast and effortlessly, and the spinach provides a touch of freshness. The feta cheese lends a salty and creamy finish. This soup is excellent for a light lunch or a big supper.

Preparation Time: 15 minutes
Cooking Time: 35 minutes
Total Time: 50 minutes

Ingredients:

- 1 tablespoon olive oil
- 1 onion, chopped
- 2 cloves garlic, minced
- 1 teaspoon ground cumin
- 1/2 teaspoon ground coriander
- 1/4 teaspoon ground turmeric
- 1/4 teaspoon salt
- 1/4 teaspoon black pepper
- 1 cup red lentils, washed and drained

- 6 cups vegetable broth
- 1 (10-ounce) container frozen spinach, thawed and squeezed dry
- 1/4 cup minced fresh parsley
- 1/4 cup crumbled feta cheese

Instructions:

- Heat the olive oil in a big saucepan over medium heat. Add the onion and garlic and simmer until softened, approximately 5 minutes.
- Add the cumin, coriander, turmeric, salt, and pepper and simmer for 1 minute longer.
- Add the lentils and stock and bring to a boil. Reduce heat to low, cover, and simmer for 20 minutes, or until the lentils are cooked.
- Stir in the spinach and parsley and simmer for 5 minutes longer, or until the spinach has wilted.
- Serve hot, topped with feta cheese.

Nutritional facts per serving:

Serving size: 6

- Calories: 320
- Carbohydrates: 40 grams
- Fat: 10 grams
- Protein: 15 grams
- Fiber: 10 grams

Tips

- For a richer soup, mash some of the lentils with a fork before serving.
- Add a dash of lemon juice or vinegar for a tangy taste.
- Garnish with more parsley or chopped fresh dill.

7. Escarole & White Bean Salad with Swordfish

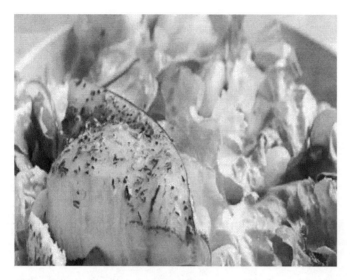

This dish is a tasty and nutritious way to eat swordfish. The fish is pan-seared and served over a bed of escarole and white bean salad with a lemon-Dijon vinaigrette. The salad is light and delicious, and the swordfish is wonderfully grilled. This meal is excellent for a light lunch or supper.

Preparation Time: 15 minutes
Cooking Time: 10 minutes
Total Time: 25 minutes

Ingredients:

- 2 10-ounce swordfish steaks
- 1 15-ounce can white beans, washed
- 1 teaspoon de Provence
- 12 cups chopped escarole
- ¼ cup very thinly sliced red onion
- ¼ cup extra-virgin olive oil
- 2 teaspoons lemon juice
- 1 teaspoon Dijon mustard

- ¼ teaspoon salt
- ¼ teaspoon powdered pepper

Instructions:

- Preheat the oven to broil.
- Whisk together the olive oil, lemon juice, mustard, salt, and pepper in a large bowl.
- Add the white beans to the dressing and toss to coat.
- Cut each swordfish steak in half so you have 4 equal servings. Sprinkle the fish with herbes de Provence and the remaining salt and pepper.
- Place the fish on a baking pan and broil for 8-10 minutes, or until just cooked through.
- While the fish is cooking, combine the escarole and red onion with the white bean salad.
- Serve the salad with the swordfish, drizzled with the remaining dressing.

Nutrition facts per serving:

Serving size: 4

- Calories: 375
- Carbohydrates: 25 grams
- Fat: 15 grams
- Protein: 35 grams
- Fiber: 10 grams

Tips

- For a more delicious salad, you may toast the escarole before adding it to the dressing.
- If you don't have herbes de Provence, you may use a blend of dried thyme, rosemary, and oregano.
- You may also serve this salad with a side of crusty bread or grilled pita bread.

8. Rainbow Grain Bowl with Cashew Tahini Sauce

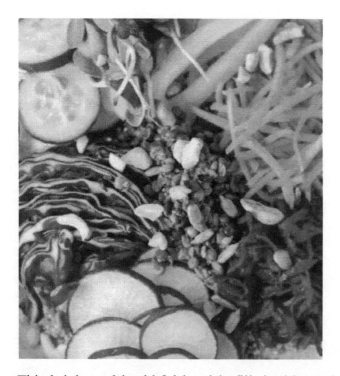

This bright and healthful bowl is filled with nutrients and makes a fantastic meal for lunch or supper. It's created with cooked lentils, quinoa, and a variety of veggies, all topped with a creamy cashew tahini sauce. The sauce is produced with only a few basic ingredients and may be easily modified to your desire.

Preparation Time: 10 minutes
Cooking Time: 0 minutes
Total Time: 10 minutes

Ingredients:

- ¾ cup unsalted cashews
- ½ cup water
- ¼ cup packed parsley leaves
- 1 tablespoon lemon juice or cider vinegar
- 1 tablespoon extra-virgin olive oil

- ½ teaspoon reduced-sodium tamari or soy sauce
- ¼ teaspoon salt
- ½ cup cooked lentils
- ½ cup cooked quinoa
- ½ cup shredded red cabbage
- ¼ cup grated raw beet
- ¼ cup chopped bell pepper
- ¼ cup shredded carrot
- ¼ cup sliced cucumber
- 1 tablespoon toasted chopped cashews (optional)

Instructions:

- Blend the cashews, water, parsley, lemon juice, olive oil, tamari, and salt in a blender until smooth.
- Place the lentils and quinoa in a small serving dish. Top with the cabbage, beet, bell pepper, carrot, and cucumber.
- Spoon 2 teaspoons of the cashew sauce over the top of each bowl.
- Garnish with toasted chopped cashews, if preferred.

Nutrition:

Serving Size: 4 servings

- Calories: 360.9
- Carbohydrates: 53.9 grams
- Fat: 10.1 grams
- Protein: 16.6 grams
- Fiber: 9.3 grams

Tips

- For a deeper taste, roast the cashews before mixing.
- To create the cashew sauce ahead of time, put it in an airtight jar in the refrigerator for up to 3 days.
- This recipe is readily adjusted to your preference. You may add or delete veggies, or use other kinds of grains.

9. Pepper Shrimp with Creamy Pecorino Oats

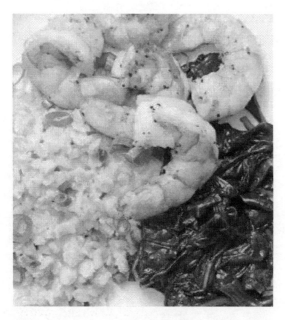

This dish is a great and quick way to have shrimp and oats for supper. The oats are cooked with scallions and pecorino cheese for a savory, creamy meal that is evocative of risotto. The shrimp are cooked in a skillet with red and green peppers, and then added to the oats. The meal is completed with a squeeze of lemon juice.

Preparation Time: 10 minutes
Cooking Time: 25 minutes
Total Time: 35 minutes

Ingredients:

- 1 cup old-fashioned oats
- 1/2 cup water
- 1/4 cup chicken broth
- 1/4 cup grated pecorino cheese 2 scallions, thinly sliced
- 1/4 teaspoon salt
- 1/8 teaspoon black pepper
- 1 pound shrimp, peeled and deveined
- 1/4 cup olive oil
- 1 red bell pepper, chopped
- 1 green bell pepper, diced
- 1 lemon, juiced

Instructions:

- In a medium saucepan, mix the oats, water, broth, pecorino cheese, scallions, salt, and pepper. Bring to a boil, then decrease heat to low and simmer for 15 minutes, or until the oats are soft.
- Meanwhile, heat the olive oil in a large pan over medium heat. Add the shrimp and heat for 2-3 minutes each side, or until pink and cooked through.
- Add the red and green peppers to the pan and simmer for 2-3 minutes, or until softened.
- Stir the shrimp and peppers into the oats. Drizzle with the lemon juice and serve immediately.

Nutritional information:

Serving size: 4

- Calories: 400
- Carbohydrates: 40 grams

- Fat: 15 grams
- Protein: 30 grams
- Fiber: 5 grams

Tips

- For a hotter meal, add a sprinkle of red pepper flakes to the oats.
- If you don't have pecorino cheese, you may use Parmesan cheese.
- Serve the meal with a side of crusty bread for dipping.

10. Pistachio-Crusted Chicken with Warm Barley Salad

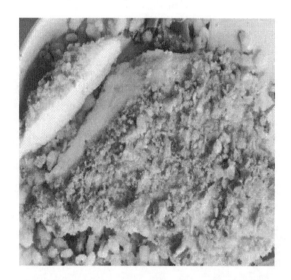

This recipe for Pistachio-Crusted Chicken with Warm Barley Salad is a great and nutritious way to have a substantial lunch. The chicken is wrapped in a crispy pistachio shell, while the barley salad is created with fresh tomatoes, parsley, and a dash of white wine vinegar. This meal is quick to prepare and can be on the table in about 30 minutes.

Preparation Time: 15 minutes
Cooking Time: 15 minutes
Total Time: 30 minutes

Ingredients:

- 2 (8 ounce) boneless, skinless chicken breasts, trimmed and split in half crosswise
- 1/2 cup salted shelled pistachios, split
- 1 teaspoon orange zest
- 1/2 cup whole-wheat panko breadcrumbs
- 1 big egg white
- 1/2 teaspoon salt, divided
- 2 tablespoons extra-virgin olive oil
- 1 cup cherry tomatoes, halved
- 1 tablespoon white-wine vinegar
- 1 cup chopped fresh parsley
- 1 cup quick barley
- 1 tablespoon water

Instructions:

- Preheat the oven to 400 degrees F (200 degrees C).
- In a food processor, pulse 1/4 cup pistachios, orange zest, and breadcrumbs until finely crushed.
- In a small dish, mix together egg white and 1/4 teaspoon salt.
- Dip chicken in egg mixture, then coat in pistachio mixture.
- Place chicken on a baking sheet coated with cooking spray.
- Bake in a preheated oven for 15 minutes, or until chicken is cooked through.
- Meanwhile, heat olive oil in a large pan over medium heat.
- Add tomatoes and vinegar to the skillet. Cook for 1 minute, or until tomatoes start to crumble.
- Stir in remaining 1/4 cup pistachios, 1/4 teaspoon salt, and parsley.
- Drain barley, if required, and incorporate into the tomato mixture.
- Serve chicken with barley salad.

Nutritional information:

Serving size: 4

- Calories: 420
- Carbohydrates: 40 grams
- Fat: 16 grams
- Protein: 30 grams
- Fiber: 5 grams

11. Acai Berry Bowl with Almond Butter

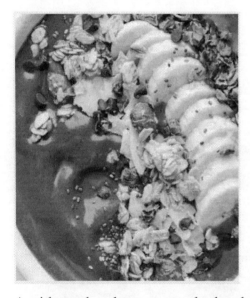

Acai berry bowls are a popular breakfast or snack choice that are filled with nutrients. They are created with a foundation of frozen acai puree, which is a high source of antioxidants, fiber, and vitamins. The acai puree is then combined with additional ingredients, such as fruit, almond butter, and granola, to make a delightful and healthful bowl.

Preparation Time: 5 minutes
Cooking Time: 0 minutes
Total Time: 5 minutes

Ingredients:

- 1 package (100g) frozen acai puree
- 1/2 cup frozen blueberries
- 1/2 cup frozen raspberries
- 1 tbsp almond butter
- 1/4 cup granola
- Toppings of your choosing, such as sliced banana, shredded coconut, chia seeds, or honey

Instructions:

- In a blender, mix the acai puree, blueberries, raspberries, almond butter, and granola. Blend until smooth.
- Pour the acai mixture into a bowl and top with your preferred toppings.

Nutritional facts (per serving):

Serving size: 1 dish

- Calories: 300
- Carbohydrates: 40 grams
- Fat: 10 grams
- Protein: 8 grams
- Fiber: 10 grams

Tips

- For a richer acai bowl, add a couple ice cubes to the blender.
- If you don't have a blender, you may crush the acai puree with a fork and then toss in the remaining ingredients.
- Feel free to experiment with various toppings to discover your favorite combo.

12. Salmon with Roasted Pepper Quinoa Salad

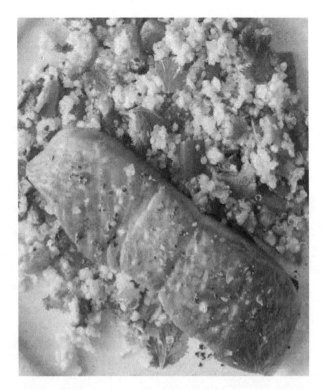

Berry Chicken Salad is a delightful and refreshing salad that is excellent for a summer meal or picnic. It is created with cooked chicken, fresh berries, and a creamy dressing. This salad is simple to cook and may be tweaked to your desire.

Preparation Time: 10 minutes
Cooking Time: 0 minutes
Total Time: 10 minutes

Ingredients:

- 2 cups cooked chicken, shredded
- 1 cup fresh berries (strawberries, blueberries, raspberries, etc.)
- 1/2 cup mayonnaise
- 1/4 cup honey
- 2 teaspoons lemon juice

- 1 teaspoon Dijon mustard
- 1/2 teaspoon salt
- 1/4 teaspoon black pepper

Instructions:

- In a large bowl, mix the chicken, berries, mayonnaise, honey, lemon juice, Dijon mustard, salt, and pepper.
- Stir until completely blended.
- Serve on toast, lettuce leaves, or crackers.

Nutritional information:

Serving size: 4 servings

- Calories: 300
- Carbohydrates: 20 grams
- Fat: 15 grams
- Protein: 20 grams
- Fiber: 5 grams

Tips

- For a healthy variation, add low-fat mayonnaise and honey.
- You may also add additional fruits to the salad, such as bananas, grapes, or peaches.
- To create the salad ahead of time, keep it in the refrigerator for up to 3 days.

13. Toast with avocado and eggs

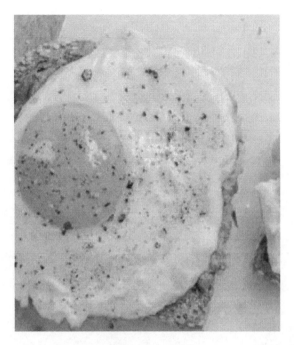

Avocado toast with eggs is a quick and simple breakfast that is both tasty and healthful. The avocado delivers healthful fats, fiber, and vitamins, while the eggs contribute protein. This dish is easy to create and may be tweaked to your desire.

Preparation Time: 5 minutes
Cooking Time: 5 minutes
Total Time: 10 minutes

Ingredients:

- 1 piece healthy grain bread
- ¼ avocado, mashed
- 1 big egg, cooked to your satisfaction
- Salt and pepper to taste
- Optional toppings: Sriracha, spicy sauce, red pepper flakes, onions, etc.

Instructions:

- Toast the bread.
- Mash the avocado with a fork or in a small bowl.
- Season the avocado with salt and pepper to taste.
- Top the bread with the mashed avocado.
- Cook the egg to your taste.
- Place the cooked egg on top of the avocado.
- Season with extra salt and pepper to taste.
- Top with your favorite optional toppings.

Nutritional Information (per serving):

Serving Size: 1 slice

- Calories: 300
- Carbohydrates: 25 grams
- Fat: 15 grams
- Protein: 10 grams
- Fiber: 5 grams

Tips

- Use your preferred kind of bread.
- Experiment with various methods to cook the egg.
- Add your favorite toppings.
- This dish can easily be doubled or tripled to satisfy a crowd.

14. Peanut butter and jelly sandwich on whole-wheat bread

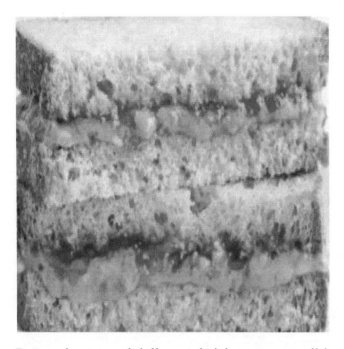

Peanut butter and jelly sandwiches are a traditional lunchbox staple that are appreciated by youngsters and adults alike. They are simple to prepare, portable, and filled with nutrients. This dish utilizes whole-wheat bread, which offers additional fiber and protein.

Preparation Time: 5 minutes

Cooking Time: 0 minutes

Total Time: 5 minutes

Ingredients:

- 4 slices whole-wheat bread
- 2 tablespoons creamy or crunchy peanut butter
- 2 tablespoons grape or strawberry jelly

Instructions:

- Spread peanut butter on one side of each piece of bread.

- Spread jelly on the opposite side of each piece of bread.
- Put the two slices together, peanut butter and jelly sides facing each other.
- Cut the sandwiches in half, if desired.

Nutritional Information:

Serving Size: 1 sandwich

- Calories: 310
- Carbohydrates: 45 grams
- Fat: 14 grams
- Protein: 8 grams
- Fiber: 5 grams

Tips

- For a healthier alternative, use natural peanut butter.
- Add a layer of banana or honey to your sandwich for added sweetness.
- Cut off the crusts to make your sandwich smaller.

Delicious Dinner Recipes

1. Fish tacos with cabbage slaw

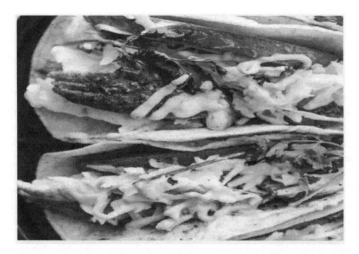

Fish tacos are a wonderful and popular Mexican delicacy. They are created with grilled or fried fish, cabbage slaw, and a variety of toppings. This recipe is for a simple and easy-to-make version of fish tacos that is excellent for a weekday supper.

Preparation Time: 15 minutes

Cooking Time: 15 minutes

Total Time: 30 minutes

Ingredients:

- 1 pound white fish filets, such as cod, halibut, or tilapia
- 1/2 teaspoon salt
- 1/4 teaspoon black pepper
- 1 tablespoon olive oil
- 1/2 cup shredded cabbage
- 1/4 cup chopped red onion
- 1/4 cup chopped cilantro

- 2 teaspoons lime juice
- 1 tablespoon mayonnaise
- 1/2 teaspoon honey
- 12 corn tortillas

Instructions:

- Preheat the oven to 400 degrees F (200 degrees C).
- Season the fish with salt and pepper.
- Heat the olive oil in a large pan over medium heat.
- Add the fish to the skillet and cook for 3-4 minutes each side, or until cooked through.
- While the fish is cooking, create the cabbage slaw. In a medium bowl, mix the cabbage, red onion, cilantro, lime juice, mayonnaise, and honey. Toss to blend.
- To create the tacos, lay a fish filet in a tortilla and top with cabbage slaw. Serve immediately.

Nutritional information:

Serving size: 2 tacos

- Calories: 370
- Carbohydrates: 23 grams
- Fat: 18 grams
- Protein: 28 grams
- Fiber: 4 grams

Tips

- For a healthy alternative, you may grill the fish instead of frying it.
- If you don't have cabbage slaw mix, you may create your own by shredding a head of cabbage.
- You may add extra toppings to your tacos, such as shredded cheese, sour cream, or avocado.

2. Turkey burgers with sweet potato fries

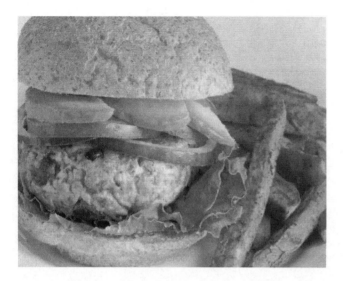

These turkey burgers with sweet potato fries are a tasty and healthful dish that is excellent for a midweek supper. The turkey burgers are seasoned with a basic combination of spices, and the sweet potato fries are crunchy and tasty. This dish is simple to follow and can be done in about an hour.

Preparation Time: 15 minutes

Cooking Time: 30 minutes

Total Time: 45 minutes

Ingredients:

For the turkey burgers:

- 1 pound ground turkey
- 1/2 onion, chopped
- 1 clove garlic, minced
- 1 teaspoon dried oregano
- 1/2 teaspoon salt
- 1/4 teaspoon black pepper

For the sweet potato fries:

- 1 big sweet potato, peeled and cut into fries
- 2 tablespoons olive oil
- 1 teaspoon smoked paprika
- 1/2 teaspoon salt
- 1/4 teaspoon black pepper

Instructions:

- Preheat the oven to 425 degrees F (220 degrees C).
- In a large bowl, mix the ground turkey, onion, garlic, oregano, salt, and pepper. Mix thoroughly to mix.
- Form the turkey mixture into 4 equal-sized patties.
- Place the sweet potato fries on a baking sheet and mix with the olive oil, smoked paprika, salt, and pepper.
- Bake the sweet potato fries for 20-25 minutes, or until golden brown and crispy.
- Heat a large skillet over medium heat.
- Add the turkey burgers to the pan and cook for 5-7 minutes each side, or until cooked through.
- Serve the turkey burgers on buns with the sweet potato fries and your preferred toppings.

Nutrition:

Serving size: 4 burgers

- Calories: 470
- Carbohydrates: 46 grams
- Fat: 21 grams
- Protein: 30 grams
- Fiber: 11 grams

Tips

- For super crispy sweet potato fries, soak them in cold water for at least one hour before frying.
- You may alternatively cook the turkey burgers on the grill or in the oven.
- Serve the turkey burgers with your favorite toppings, such as lettuce, tomato, avocado, or cheese.

3. Veggie burgers with quinoa salad

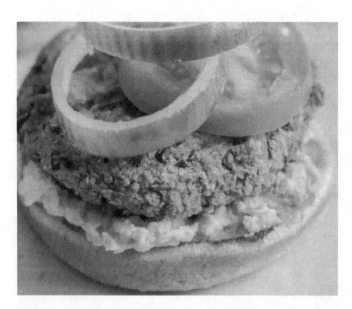

These vegetarian burgers with quinoa salad are a tasty and comforting dish that is suitable for a summer BBQ or a weekday supper. The burgers are created with a healthy blend of quinoa, black beans, veggies, and spices, and they are grilled till golden brown and crispy. The quinoa salad is a pleasant side dish that is created with quinoa, cucumbers, tomatoes, and a mild vinaigrette dressing.

Preparation Time: 15 minutes
Cooking Time: 15 minutes
Total Time: 30 minutes

Ingredients:

For the vegetarian burgers:

- 1 cup cooked quinoa
- 1 (15-ounce) can black beans, washed and drained
- 1/2 cup chopped onion
- 1/2 cup chopped red bell pepper
- 1/4 cup breadcrumbs
- 1 egg, beaten
- 1 tablespoon ground cumin
- 1 teaspoon chili powder
- 1/2 teaspoon salt
- 1/4 teaspoon black pepper

For the quinoa salad:

- 1 cup cooked quinoa
- 1/2 cup chopped cucumber
- 1/2 cup chopped tomato
- 1/4 cup chopped red onion
- 2 tablespoons olive oil
- 2 tablespoons balsamic vinegar
- 1 teaspoon salt
- 1/4 teaspoon black pepper

Instructions:

To make the vegetarian burgers:

- In a large bowl, mix the cooked quinoa, black beans, onion, bell pepper, breadcrumbs, egg, cumin, chili powder, salt, and pepper. Mix vigorously until the ingredients are uniformly blended.
- Form the mixture into 4 patties, approximately 4 inches in diameter.
- Heat a large skillet over medium heat. Add a drizzle of olive oil to the pan.
- Cook the vegetable burgers for 3-4 minutes each side, or until golden brown and cooked through.

To create the quinoa salad:

- In a large bowl, add the cooked quinoa, cucumber, tomato, red onion, olive oil, balsamic vinegar, salt, and pepper. Mix vigorously until the ingredients are uniformly blended.

To serve:

- Serve the vegetarian burgers on buns with your favorite toppings, such as lettuce, tomato, avocado, and your favorite sauce. Serve the quinoa salad on the side.

Nutrition per serving:

Serving size: 4 vegetarian burgers, 1 quinoa salad

- Calories: 470
- Carbohydrates: 55 grams
- Fat: 15 grams
- Protein: 25 grams
- Fiber: 10 grams

4. Black bean soup with cornbread

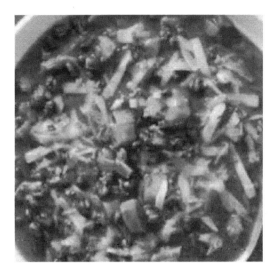

This thick and fragrant black bean soup is a delightful and wholesome supper. It is a wonderful source of protein, fiber, and complex carbs. The cornbread provides a hint of sweetness and maize flavor that wonderfully compliments the soup. This dish is simple to create and may be easily tweaked to your desire.

Preparation Time: 15 minutes
Cooking Time: 20 minutes
Total Time: 35 minutes

Ingredients:

- 1 tablespoon olive oil
- 1 onion, chopped
- 2 cloves garlic, minced
- 1 teaspoon chili powder
- 1/2 teaspoon cumin
- 1/4 teaspoon cayenne pepper
- 1 (15-ounce) can black beans, washed and drained
- 1 (15-ounce) can corn, drained

- 4 cups vegetable broth
- Salt and pepper to taste

Instructions:

- Heat the olive oil in a big saucepan over medium heat. Add the onion and garlic and simmer until softened, approximately 5 minutes.
- Add the chili powder, cumin, and cayenne pepper and simmer for 1 minute longer.
- Stir in the black beans, corn, vegetable broth, salt, and pepper. Bring to a boil, then decrease heat and simmer for 20 minutes, or until the flavors have merged.
- Serve hot with cornbread.

Nutritional information:

Serving size: 6 servings

- Calories: 230
- Carbohydrates: 40 grams
- Fat: 7 grams
- Protein: 12 grams
- Fiber: 12 grams

Tips

- For a richer soup, purée some of the beans in a blender before adding them to the saucepan.
- Add your favorite toppings, such as shredded cheese, sour cream, or avocado.
- This soup may be prepared ahead of time and kept in the refrigerator for up to 3 days.

5. Tofu scramble

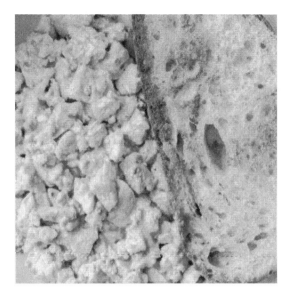

Tofu scramble is a vegan meal that is produced by scrambling tofu in a skillet with spices and veggies. It is a terrific way to use up surplus tofu and is a nutritious and fulfilling breakfast or brunch alternative.

Preparation Time: 10 minutes

Cooking Time: 15 minutes

Total Time: 25 minutes

Ingredients:

- 1 block extra-firm tofu, drained and pressed
- 1 tablespoon olive oil
- 1/2 onion, chopped
- 1 clove garlic, minced
- 1 teaspoon turmeric powder
- 1/2 teaspoon ground cumin
- 1/4 teaspoon salt
- 1/4 teaspoon black pepper

- 1/4 cup nutritional yeast
- 1/4 cup vegetable broth

Instructions:

- Heat the olive oil in a large pan over medium heat.
- Crumble the tofu into the pan and cook, turning constantly, for 5 minutes, or until the tofu is browned.
- Add the onion and garlic to the skillet and heat, turning periodically, for 5 minutes, or until the onion is softened.
- Stir in the turmeric powder, cumin, salt, and black pepper. Cook for 1 minute, or until aromatic.
- Stir in the nutritional yeast and vegetable broth.
- Cook for 2 minutes, or until the sauce has thickened.
- Serve immediately.

Nutrition:

Serving size: 4 servings

- Calories: 250
- Carbohydrates: 15 grams
- Fat: 15 grams
- Protein: 15 grams
- Fiber: 5 grams

Tips

- For a creamier scramble, add 1/4 cup of mashed avocado or vegan yogurt.
- For a hotter scramble, add 1/4 teaspoon of cayenne pepper or red pepper flakes.
- Serve the scramble with your favorite toppings, such as fresh salsa, avocado, or vegan cheese.

6. Pasta with roasted veggies

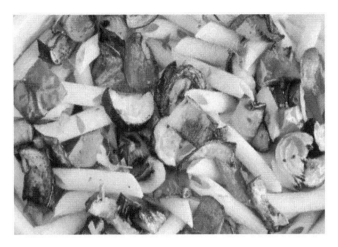

Pasta with roasted veggies is a tasty and healthful recipe that is excellent for a midweek supper. The roasted veggies lend a hint of sweetness and smokiness to the pasta, and the entire meal is done in under an hour.

Preparation Time: 15 minutes

Cooking Time: 30 minutes

Total Time: 45 minutes

Ingredients:

- 1 pound spaghetti of your choice
- 1 tablespoon olive oil
- 1 onion, chopped
- 2 carrots, chopped
- 1 zucchini, chopped
- 1 red bell pepper, chopped
- 1 (14.5 ounce) can diced tomatoes, undrained
- 1 teaspoon dried oregano
- 1/2 teaspoon salt
- 1/4 teaspoon black pepper

Instructions:

- Preheat the oven to 400 degrees F (200 degrees C).
- Toss veggies with olive oil, oregano, salt, and pepper.
- Spread veggies on a baking sheet and roast for 25-30 minutes, or until soft and slightly browned.
- Meanwhile, prepare pasta according to package instructions.
- Drain pasta and add to a large bowl.
- Stir in roasted veggies and chopped tomatoes.
- Serve immediately.

Nutrition:

Serving Size: 4 persons

- Calories: 450
- Carbohydrates: 60 grams
- Fat: 10 grams
- Protein: 15 grams
- Fiber: 5 grams

Tips

- You may use whatever sort of pasta you prefer for this recipe.
- If you don't have dry oregano, you may use 1/2 teaspoon of fresh oregano.
- You may also add additional veggies to this dish, such as mushrooms, eggplant, or spinach.
- For a more delicious dinner, you may roast the veggies in a blend of olive oil and balsamic vinegar.
- Serve this meal with a side of crusty bread or a green salad.

7. Pasta with marinara sauce

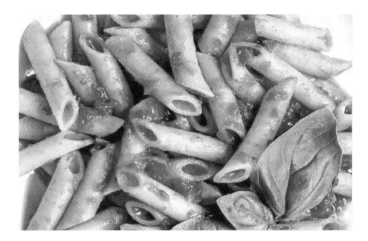

Pasta with marinara sauce is a traditional Italian meal that is simple to prepare and always a crowd-pleaser. The sauce is created with basic components like tomatoes, garlic, and herbs, and it is cooked until it is thick and tasty. The pasta is cooked al dente and then mixed with the sauce. This recipe is excellent for a fast and simple weekday supper, or for a more formal dinner gathering.

Preparation Time: 15 minutes
Cooking Time: 20 minutes
Total Time: 35 minutes

Ingredients:

- 1 tablespoon olive oil
- 4 cloves garlic, minced
- 1 (28-ounce) can crushed tomatoes
- 1 teaspoon dried oregano
- 1/2 teaspoon salt
- 1/4 teaspoon black pepper
- 1 pound dry pasta
- Grated Parmesan cheese, for serving (optional)

Instructions:

- Heat the olive oil in a big saucepan over medium heat. Add the garlic and sauté until fragrant, approximately 1 minute.
- Add the smashed tomatoes, oregano, salt, and pepper to the pot. Bring to a boil and cook for 20 minutes, or until the sauce has thickened.
- While the sauce is boiling, cook the pasta according to the package instructions.
- Drain the pasta and add it to the sauce. Toss to coat.
- Serve immediately, with grated Parmesan cheese, if preferred.

Nutrition:

Serving size: 4

- Calories: 350
- Carbohydrates: 50 grams
- Fat: 10 grams
- Protein: 15 grams
- Fiber: 5 grams

Variations:

- Add some chopped veggies to the sauce, such as carrots, onions, or peppers.
- For a heartier meal, add some cooked ground beef or sausage to the sauce.
- Serve the spaghetti with a side of crusty bread or garlic toast.

Tips

- If you don't have dried oregano, you may use 1/2 teaspoon of dried basil.
- If you want a smoother sauce, you may purée it in a blender or food processor.
- If you prefer a hotter sauce, add a sprinkle of red pepper flakes.

8. Lentil stew with brown rice

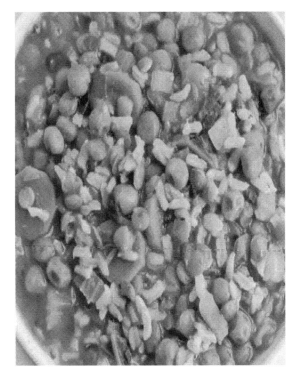

Lentil stew with brown rice is a substantial and healthy dinner that is excellent for a chilly winter day. It is rich with protein, fiber, and complex carbs, making it a substantial and fulfilling meal. This dish is also vegan and gluten-free, so it may be enjoyed by individuals with dietary requirements.

Preparation Time: 15 minutes
Cooking Time: 30 minutes
Total Time: 45 minutes

Ingredients:

- 1 tablespoon olive oil
- 1 onion, chopped
- 2 carrots, chopped
- 2 celery stalks, chopped

- 2 cloves garlic, minced
- 1 teaspoon dried thyme
- 1/2 teaspoon ground cumin
- 1/4 teaspoon salt
- 1/4 teaspoon black pepper
- 1 cup brown rice
- 1 cup lentils, washed and drained
- 4 cups vegetable broth
- 1 bay leaf
- 1/2 cup chopped fresh parsley

Instructions:

- Heat the olive oil in a big saucepan over medium heat. Add the onion, carrots, celery, and garlic and simmer until softened, approximately 5 minutes.
- Add the thyme, cumin, salt, and pepper and simmer for 1 minute longer.
- Stir in the brown rice, lentils, vegetable broth, and bay leaf. Bring to a boil, then decrease heat to low, cover, and simmer for 30 minutes, or until the rice and lentils are cooked through.
- Stir in the parsley and serve.

Nutritional facts per serving:

Serving size: 6

- Calories: 375
- Carbohydrates: 50 grams
- Fat: 10 grams
- Protein: 15 grams
- Fiber: 15 grams

Tips

- For a deeper taste, you may sauté the lentils in a separate skillet before adding them to the stew.

- If you don't have vegetable broth, you may substitute water or chicken broth.

- To prepare this stew ahead of time, cook it according to the directions, then let it cool fully. Store it in the refrigerator for up to 3 days or in the freezer for up to 3 months. When you're ready to eat, reheat it over low heat until warmed through.

9. Tomato Soup

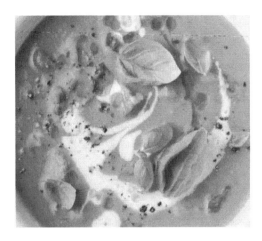

Tomato soup is a traditional comfort dish that is simple to prepare and always a success. This recipe is basic and uncomplicated, but it yields a thick and savory soup that is excellent for a chilly winter day.

Preparation Time: 15 minutes
Cooking Time: 30 minutes
Total Time: 45 minutes

Ingredients:

- 1 tablespoon olive oil
- 1/2 onion, chopped

- 2 cloves garlic, minced
- 1 (28-ounce) can crushed tomatoes, undrained
- 1 (14.5-ounce) can chopped tomatoes, undrained
- 1 teaspoon dried oregano
- 1/2 teaspoon salt
- 1/4 teaspoon black pepper
- 1/2 cup chicken broth
- 1/4 cup heavy cream
- 1/4 cup grated Parmesan cheese

Instructions:

- Heat the olive oil in a big saucepan over medium heat. Add the onion and garlic and simmer until softened, approximately 5 minutes. 2. Stir in the crushed tomatoes, diced tomatoes, oregano, salt, and pepper. Bring to a boil, then decrease heat and simmer for 20 minutes, or until the flavors have merged.
- Stir in the chicken broth and cream and bring to a boil. Cook for another 5 minutes, or until heated through.
- Puree the soup in a blender or food processor until smooth.
- Stir in the Parmesan cheese and serve.

Nutritional information:

Serving size: 6 servings

- Calories: 230
- Carbohydrates: 30 grams
- Fat: 10 grams
- Protein: 6 grams
- Fiber: 5 grams

Tips

- For a richer soup, add an extra 1/4 cup of heavy cream.
- For a healthy soup, use low-sodium chicken broth and fat-free half-and-half.
- Garnish the soup with a dollop of sour cream, croutons, or grated Parmesan cheese.

10. Lentil Soup

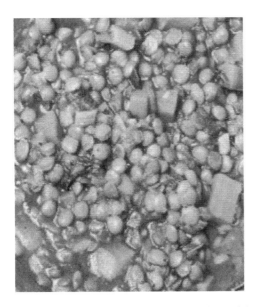

Lentil soup is a substantial and healthy soup that is cooked with lentils, veggies, and stock. It is an excellent source of protein, fiber, and other nutrients. This dish is simple to create and may be tweaked to your desire.

Preparation Time: 15 minutes
Cooking Time: 30-40 minutes
Total Time: 45-60 minutes

Ingredients:

- 2 tablespoons olive oil
- 1 onion, chopped
- 2 carrots, chopped

- 2 celery stalks, chopped
- 2 cloves garlic, minced
- 1 teaspoon dried thyme
- 1 teaspoon ground cumin
- 1/2 teaspoon salt
- 1/4 teaspoon black pepper
- 2 cups dry lentils, washed and sorted
- 6 cups vegetable broth
- 1/2 cup chopped fresh parsley

Instructions:

- Heat the olive oil in a big saucepan over medium heat. Add the onion, carrots, celery, and garlic and simmer until softened, approximately 5 minutes.
- Add the thyme, cumin, salt, and pepper and simmer for 1 minute longer.
- Add the lentils and stock and bring to a boil. Reduce heat to low, cover, and simmer for 30-40 minutes, or until the lentils are cooked.
- Stir in the parsley and serve.

Nutritional facts per serving:

Serving size: 6 cups

- Calories: 300
- Carbohydrates: 45 grams
- Fat: 10 grams
- Protein: 15 grams
- Fiber: 15 grams

Tips

- You may use whatever sort of lentils you prefer in this soup.
- If you prefer a thicker soup, you may purée portions of the soup before serving.
- Serve with fresh bread or crackers for a full supper.

11. Tofu Scramble with Spinach and Peppers

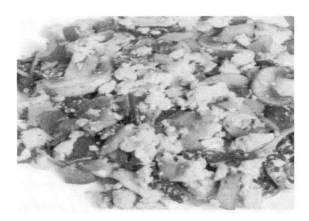

This tofu scramble is a wonderful and healthful breakfast or lunch choice. It is created with crumbled tofu, spinach, peppers, and a few basic seasonings. The scramble is simple to prepare and may be adjusted to your desire.

Preparation Time: 10 minutes
Cooking Time: 15 minutes
Total Time: 25 minutes

Ingredients:

- 1 block extra-firm tofu, drained and pressed
- 1 tablespoon olive oil
- 1/2 onion, chopped
- 1 bell pepper, chopped
- 1 cup spinach leaves
- 1 teaspoon turmeric powder

- 1/2 teaspoon salt
- 1/4 teaspoon black pepper

Instructions:

- Heat the olive oil in a large pan over medium heat.
- Add the onion and bell pepper and simmer until softened, approximately 5 minutes.
- Crumble the tofu into the pan and heat, turning periodically, until browned, approximately 10 minutes.
- Stir in the spinach, turmeric, salt, and pepper. Cook until the spinach is wilted, approximately 2 minutes.
- Serve immediately.

Nutritions:

Serving size: 4 servings

- Calories: 250
- Carbohydrates: 15 grams
- Fat: 15 grams
- Protein: 20 grams
- Fiber: 5 grams

Tips

- For a creamier scramble, add 1/4 cup of unsweetened almond milk or soy milk.
- For a hotter scramble, add 1/2 teaspoon of chili powder or cayenne pepper.
- To prepare ahead, crumble the tofu and sauté the veggies until softened. Then, put the mixture in an airtight jar in the refrigerator for up to 3 days. When you're ready to eat, just reheat the mixture in a pan over medium heat until cooked through.

12. Shrimp Scampi with Zucchini Noodles

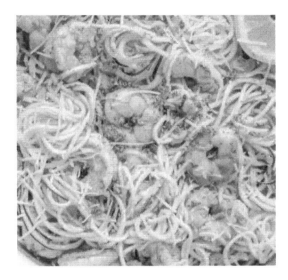

This recipe is a tasty and nutritious take on the traditional Italian meal, Shrimp Scampi. It utilizes zucchini noodles instead of regular pasta, which makes it a lower-carb and higher-fiber choice. The shrimp are cooked in a delicious sauce composed with butter, garlic, white wine, and lemon juice. The entire recipe comes together fast and simply, making it a terrific evening supper.

Preparation Time: 15 minutes

Cooking Time: 10 minutes

Total Time: 25 minutes

Ingredients:

- 1 pound zucchini, spiralized
- 1 tablespoon olive oil
- 1/4 cup butter
- 2 cloves garlic, minced
- 1/4 cup white wine
- 1/4 cup lemon juice
- 1 pound big shrimp, peeled and deveined
- Salt and pepper to taste

- 1/4 cup chopped fresh parsley

Instructions:

- Heat the olive oil in a large pan over medium heat. Add the butter and garlic and heat until fragrant, approximately 1 minute.
- Add the white wine and lemon juice and bring to a boil. Reduce heat to low and simmer for 5 minutes.
- Add the shrimp to the pan and heat until pink and cooked through, approximately 2 minutes each side. Season with salt and pepper.
- Stir in the zucchini noodles and parsley and simmer until cooked through, approximately 1 minute.
- Serve immediately.

Nutritional facts per serving:

Serving size: 4

- Calories: 340
- Carbohydrates: 14 grams
- Fat: 20 grams
- Protein: 28 grams
- Fiber: 4 grams

Tips

- You may use any sort of spiralized vegetable in this dish, such as carrots, cucumbers, or sweet potatoes.
- To spiralize zucchini, you may use a spiralizer or a vegetable peeler.
- If you don't have white wine, you may use chicken broth or vegetarian broth.
- Garnish with more parsley and lemon wedges, if preferred.

13. Salmon with Lemon and Capers

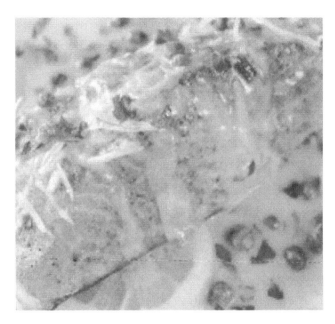

Salmon with lemon and capers is a traditional and tasty recipe that is simple to create. The salmon is cooked to perfection in a simple lemon and caper sauce, and the result is a juicy, delicious fish that is excellent for a weekday supper.

Preparation Time: 10 minutes

Cooking Time: 15 minutes

Total Time: 25 minutes

Ingredients:

- 2 (6-ounce) salmon filets, skin on 1 tablespoon olive oil
- 1/2 teaspoon salt
- 1/4 teaspoon black pepper
- 1 lemon, finely sliced
- 1 tablespoon capers, drained
- 1/4 cup dry white wine

Instructions:

- Preheat the oven to 400 degrees F (200 degrees C).
- Pat salmon filets dry with paper towels. Season with salt and pepper.
- Heat olive oil in a large pan over medium heat.
- Add salmon filets, skin side down, to the skillet. Cook for 5 minutes, or until the skin is golden brown.
- Flip the salmon filets and top with lemon slices, capers, and white wine.
- Bake in the preheated oven for 10-12 minutes, or until the salmon is cooked through.
- Serve immediately.

Nutrition:

Serving size: 2

- Calories: 400
- Carbohydrates: 10 grams
- Fat: 20 grams
- Protein: 30 grams
- Fiber: 0 grams

Tips

- For a crispier exterior, score the salmon filets with a sharp knife before cooking.
- If you don't have capers, you may substitute another salty item, such as olives or anchovies.
- Serve the salmon with your favorite sides, such as roasted veggies, rice, or pasta.

14. Quinoa Bowl with Roasted Vegetables

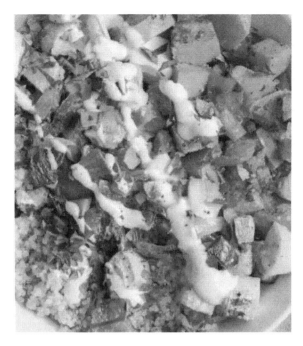

This dish is a healthy and tasty way to get your daily dose of veggies. The quinoa is a fantastic source of protein and fiber, and the roasted veggies contribute a range of vitamins and minerals. This dish is also vegan and gluten-free, making it a wonderful alternative for anyone with dietary limitations.

Preparation Time: 15 minutes

Cooking Time: 35 minutes

Total Time: 50 minutes

Ingredients:

- 1 cup quinoa, rinsed
- 1/2 cups water
- 1/2 teaspoon salt
- 1 tablespoon olive oil
- 1 onion, chopped

- 1 red bell pepper, chopped
- 1 green bell pepper, chopped
- 1 sweet potato, peeled and diced
- 1 teaspoon garlic powder
- 1/2 teaspoon salt
- 1/4 teaspoon black pepper
- Chopped parsley, for garnish (optional)

Instructions:

- In a small saucepan, mix the quinoa, water, and salt. Bring to a boil over medium heat. Reduce heat to low, cover, and simmer for 15 minutes, or until the quinoa is cooked through.
- Meanwhile, preheat the oven to 425 degrees F (220 degrees C).
- In a large bowl, add the onion, bell peppers, sweet potato, olive oil, garlic powder, salt, and pepper. Toss to coat.
- Spread the veggies on a baking sheet and roast for 20-25 minutes, or until soft and slightly browned.
- To construct the bowls, divide the quinoa into 4 bowls. Top with the roasted veggies and sprinkle with parsley, if preferred.

Nutrition:

Serving size: 1 dish

- Calories: 420
- Carbohydrates: 55 grams
- Fat: 15 grams
- Protein: 15 grams
- Fiber: 9 grams

15. Lentil Salad with Walnuts and Cranberries

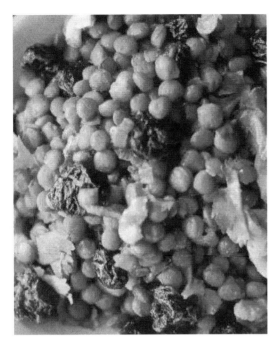

Lentil Salad with Walnuts and Cranberries is a tasty and nutritious salad that is excellent for a light meal or a healthy side dish. It is created with lentils, walnuts, cranberries, and a basic vinaigrette dressing. The salad is robust and delicious, but it is also light and refreshing.

Preparation Time: 10 minutes

Cooking Time: 25 minutes

Total Time: 35 minutes

Ingredients:

- 1 cup dry lentils, washed and drained
- 2 cups water
- 1/2 cup walnuts, toasted and chopped
- 1/2 cup dried cranberries
- 1/4 cup olive oil
- 2 teaspoons lemon juice

- 1 teaspoon honey
- 1/2 teaspoon salt
- 1/4 teaspoon black pepper

Instructions:

- Bring the lentils and water to a boil in a medium saucepan. Reduce heat to low, cover, and simmer for 20-25 minutes, or until the lentils are cooked. Drain the lentils and leave aside to cool.
- In a large bowl, mix together the olive oil, lemon juice, honey, salt, and pepper. Add the lentils, walnuts, and cranberries to the bowl and mix to coat.
- Serve the salad immediately or refrigerate for later.

Nutritional information:

Serving size: 1 cup

- Calories: 350
- Carbohydrates: 40 grams
- Fat: 15 grams
- Protein: 15 grams
- Fiber: 8 grams

Tips

- For a more delicious salad, toast the walnuts in a dry pan over medium heat for a few minutes, or until they are aromatic and lightly toasted.
- You may also add additional components to the salad, such as feta cheese, chopped red onion, or chopped fresh herbs.
- This salad is best served cold, but it may also be served at room temperature.

CHAPTER FOUR

Mouthwatering Snacks And Desserts Recipes

Snacks Recipes

1. Orange Slices

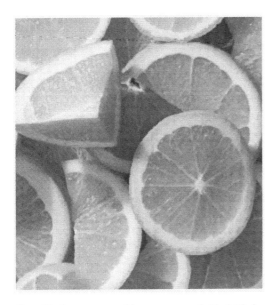

Candied orange slices are a delightful and easy-to-make delicacy that may be eaten as a snack, dessert, or garnish. They are created by cooking orange slices in a simple syrup until they are soft and transparent. The resultant slices are sweet and acidic, with a chewy texture.

Preparation Time: 15 minutes
Cooking Time: 45-60 minutes
Total Time: 1 hour

Ingredients:

- 4 big oranges

- 4 cups water
- 4 cups granulated sugar

Instructions:

- Wash the oranges and slice them into 1/4-inch thick rounds.
- In a large saucepan, mix the water and sugar. Bring to a boil over medium heat, stirring frequently until the sugar is dissolved.
- Add the orange slices to the pot and decrease heat to low. Simmer for 45-60 minutes, or until the orange slices are soft and transparent.
- Remove the orange slices from the syrup and let cool on a wire rack.

Nutrition:

Serving Size: 24 orange slices

- Calories: 100
- Carbohydrates: 25 grams
- Fat: 0 grams
- Protein: 1 gram
- Fiber: 1 gram

Tips

- For a fuller taste, use a blend of white and brown sugar.
- To avoid the orange slices from adhering to the bottom of the saucepan, place a tiny piece of parchment paper to the bottom before adding the slices.
- If you wish to dry the orange slices, put them on a wire rack in a single layer and set them in a low oven (200 degrees Fahrenheit) for 2-3 hours.

2. Kale Chips

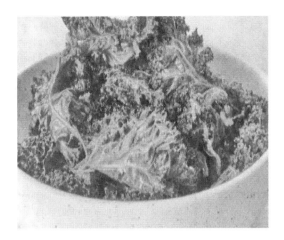

Kale chips are a nutritious and tasty snack that can be produced in just a few minutes. They are a fantastic source of vitamins A, C, and K, and they are also low in calories and fat.

Preparation Time: 10 minutes

Cooking Time: 20-25 minutes

Total Time: 30-35 minutes

Ingredients:

- 1 huge bunch of kale, cleaned and dried
- 1 tablespoon olive oil
- 1/2 teaspoon salt
- 1/4 teaspoon black pepper
- Other alternative ingredients, such as garlic powder, onion powder, or chili powder

Instructions:

- Preheat the oven to 300 degrees F (150 degrees C).
- Remove the stems from the kale leaves and break the leaves into bite-sized pieces.
- In a large bowl, combine the kale leaves with the olive oil, salt, and pepper.

- Spread the kale leaves in a single layer on a baking sheet coated with parchment paper.
- Bake for 20-25 minutes, or until the kale leaves are crispy.
- Let the kale chips cool fully before serving.

Nutrition:

Serving size: 4 servings of kale chips

- Calories: 120
- Carbohydrates: 15 grams
- Fat: 10 grams
- Protein: 3 grams
- Fiber: 5 grams

Tips

- To make sure the kale chips are crispy, make sure they are spread out in a single layer on the baking pan.
- If you want to add extra flavor to the kale chips, you may add other spices, such as garlic powder, onion powder, or chili powder.
- You may also add various varieties of kale to the dish, such as curly kale or red kale.
- Kale chips may be kept in an airtight jar at room temperature for up to 3 days.

3. Frozen Grapes

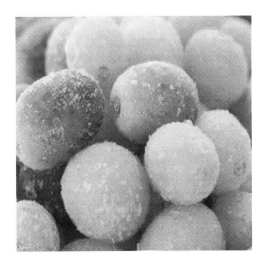

Frozen grapes are a delightful and healthful snack that is suitable for any time of year. They are low in calories and fat, and they are a wonderful source of vitamins and minerals. Frozen grapes may be consumed on their own, or they can be added to smoothies, yogurt, or salads.

Preparation Time: 10 minutes

Cooking Time: 0 minutes

Total Time: 10 minutes

Ingredients:

- 1 pound grapes, washed and stemmed

Instructions:

- Rinse the grapes in cool water and remove the stems.
- Place the grapes in a single layer on a baking sheet or platter.
- Freeze the grapes for at least 8 hours, preferably overnight.
- Enjoy!

Nutritional facts per serving:

Serving size: 1 cup

- Calories: 70
- Carbohydrates: 15 grams
- Fat: 0 grams
- Protein: 1 gram
- Fiber: 2 grams

Tips

- You may freeze grapes in various colors for a fun and colorful snack.
- Frozen grapes may also be used as ice cubes in beverages.
- If you want to add a little sweetness to your frozen grapes, you may toss them in a tiny quantity of sugar or honey before freezing.

4. Berries or Peach Slices with Greek Yogurt

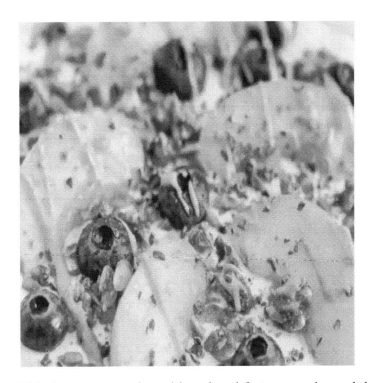

This is an easy and nutritious breakfast or snack meal that is excellent for a hot summer day. It is created with Greek yogurt, fresh berries or peaches, and your favorite toppings. The yogurt delivers protein and calcium, while the fruit adds flavor and antioxidants.

Preparation Time: 5 minutes

Cooking Time: 0 minutes

Total Time: 5 minutes

Ingredients:

- 1 cup plain Greek yogurt
- 1 cup fresh berries or peaches, sliced
- 1/4 cup granola or muesli
- 1 tablespoon honey or maple syrup (optional)

Instructions:

- In a bowl, mix the Greek yogurt, berries or peaches, granola, and honey or maple syrup (if using).
- Serve immediately.

Nutrition:

Serving size: 1 cup

- Calories: 250-300
- Carbohydrates: 30-40 grams
- Fat: 10-15 grams
- Protein: 15-20 grams
- Fiber: 5-10 grams

Tips

- You may use any sort of berries or peaches that you prefer.
- If you don't have granola, you may substitute muesli, oats, or even cereal.
- You may also add additional toppings, such as nuts, seeds, or chocolate chips.
- This recipe can easily be doubled or tripled to produce a bigger quantity.

5. Trail Mix

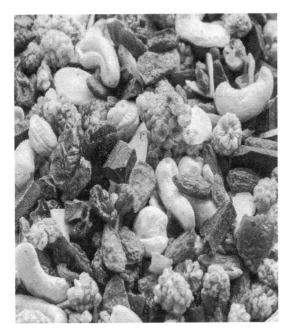

Trail mix is a tasty and nutritious snack that is excellent for hiking, camping, or simply as a fast pick-me-up. It is a blend of nuts, seeds, dried fruit, and occasionally granola. The ingredients may vary based on your tastes, but some common possibilities include almonds, cashews, peanuts, raisins, cranberries, and M&Ms.

Preparation Time: 10 minutes

Cooking Time: None

Total Time: 10 minutes

Ingredients:

- 1 cup almonds
- 1 cup cashews
- 1 cup peanuts
- 1/2 cup raisins
- 1/2 cup cranberries
- 1/4 cup granola (optional)

Instructions:

- Measure out the ingredients and mix them in a bowl.
- If you are using granola, toast it in the oven for a few minutes beforehand.
- Stir to blend the ingredients.
- Enjoy!

Nutrition:

Serving Size: The serving size for trail mix is roughly 1/2 cup

- Calories: 250
- Carbohydrates: 25 grams
- Fat: 15 grams
- Protein: 10 grams
- Fiber: 5 grams

Tips

- You may add whatever nuts and dried fruits that you prefer in trail mix.
- If you want to make your trail mix more energy-dense, you may add some chocolate chips or M&Ms.
- Trail mix is an excellent snack to take on treks or camping vacations. It is also a nutritious and enjoyable snack to keep on hand for those occasions when you need a fast pick-me-up.

6. Baked Apple Chips

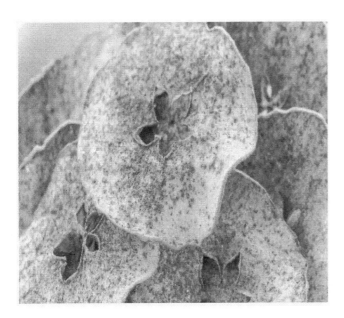

Baked apple chips are a nutritious and delightful snack that is simple to prepare. They are an excellent source of fiber, vitamin C, and antioxidants. This dish involves a basic technique of slicing apples thinly and baking them in the oven until they are crisp. You may add cinnamon or other spices to taste.

Preparation Time: 15 minutes

Cooking Time: 1 hour

Total Time: 1 hour 15 minutes

Ingredients:

- 2 big apples, peeled, cored, and thinly sliced (approximately 1/8-inch thick)
- 1 teaspoon ground cinnamon (optional)

Instructions:

- Preheat the oven to 200 degrees F (93 degrees C).
- Line two baking pans with parchment paper.

- Arrange apple slices in a single layer on the prepared baking sheets.
- Sprinkle with cinnamon, if preferred.
- Bake for 1 hour, or until the apples are crisp.
- Let cool fully on the baking sheets before storing in an airtight container.

Nutrition:

Serving size: 1/4 cup

- Calories: 75
- Carbohydrates: 15 grams
- Fat: 0 grams
- Protein: 1 gram
- Fiber: 3 grams

Tips

- For the crispiest apple chips, use a mandoline to slice the apples.
- If you don't have cinnamon, you may add other spices, such as nutmeg, ginger, or cardamom.
- You may also add dried fruit, such as cranberries or raisins, to the apple chips.
- Store apple chips in an airtight jar at room temperature for up to 1 week.

7. Carrots with Hummus

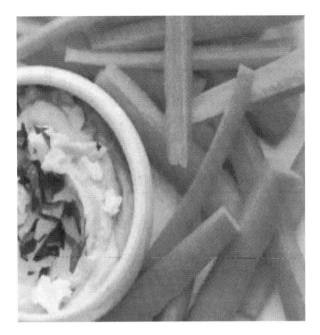

Carrots with hummus is a popular and healthful snack or light supper. The carrots are roasted till soft and slightly sweet, and the hummus is creamy and tasty. This dish is simple to prepare and only takes around 30 minutes altogether.

Preparation Time: 10 minutes

Cooking Time: 20 minutes

Total Time: 30 minutes

Ingredients:

- 1 pound carrots, peeled and cut into sticks
- 2 tablespoons olive oil
- 1/2 teaspoon salt
- 1/4 teaspoon black pepper
- 1 (15-ounce) can chickpeas, drained and rinsed
- 1/4 cup tahini
- 2 teaspoons lemon juice

- 1 clove garlic, minced
- 1/4 teaspoon salt
- 1/4 teaspoon black pepper

Instructions:

- Preheat the oven to 400 degrees F (200 degrees C).
- Toss carrots with olive oil, salt, and pepper.
- Spread carrots on a baking sheet and roast for 20-25 minutes, or until soft.
- Meanwhile, prepare the hummus: In a food processor, mix chickpeas, tahini, lemon juice, garlic, salt, and pepper. Process till smooth.
- Serve carrots with hummus.

Nutritional information:

Serving size: 1 cup carrots with 1/3 cup hummus

- Calories: 280
- Carbohydrates: 35 grams
- Fat: 12 grams
- Protein: 8 grams
- Fiber: 5 grams

Tips

- For a more delicious hummus, toast the garlic cloves before adding them to the food processor.
- Serve carrots and hummus with pita bread, crackers, or veggies.
- Store leftover hummus in an airtight jar in the refrigerator for up to 5 days.

8. Carrot and Cucumber Dip

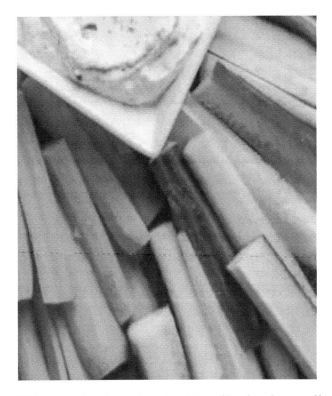

This is a simple and refreshing dip that is excellent for a healthy snack or appetizer. It is created with only a few ingredients, and it is ready in just a few minutes. The carrots and cucumbers lend a hint of sweetness and crunch, while the yogurt and lemon juice give it a tangy taste.

Preparation Time: 5 minutes

Cooking Time: 0 minutes

Total Time: 5 minutes

Ingredients:

- 1 cup grated carrots
- 1 cup grated cucumber
- 1/2 cup plain yogurt
- 1 tablespoon lemon juice
- 1 teaspoon honey

- 1/4 teaspoon salt
- 1/8 teaspoon black pepper

Instructions:

- In a medium bowl, mix the carrots, cucumber, yogurt, lemon juice, honey, salt, and pepper.
- Stir until completely blended.
- Serve immediately with your favorite dippers.

Nutrition:

Serving size: 1/2 cup

- Calories: 100
- Carbohydrates: 15 grams
- Fat: 5 grams
- Protein: 3 grams
- Fiber: 2 grams

Tips

- For a smoother dip, you may purée the carrots and cucumbers in a blender or food processor before adding them to the yogurt.
- You may also add additional ingredients to the dip, such as chopped fresh herbs, grated Parmesan cheese, or a touch of cayenne pepper.
- Store the dip in an airtight jar in the refrigerator for up to 3 days.

9. Cranberry Cashew Butter

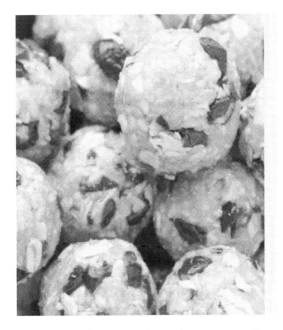

These cranberry cashew butter snacks are a tasty and nutritious way to satisfy your sweet appetite. They are prepared with basic ingredients, such cashew butter, oats, dried cranberries, and maple syrup, and they are naturally gluten-free and vegan. They are also an excellent source of protein, fiber, and healthy fats.

Preparation Time: 10 minutes
Cooking Time: 0 minutes
Total Time: 10 minutes

Ingredients:

- 1 cup old-fashioned oats
- 1/2 cup cashew butter
- 1/4 cup dried cranberries
- 2 tablespoons maple syrup
- 1/4 teaspoon salt

Instructions:

- In a food processor, mix the oats, cashew butter, cranberries, maple syrup, and salt. Process until the material is fully blended and resembles a dough.
- Roll the dough into 1-inch balls.
- Place the balls on a parchment-lined baking sheet and refrigerate for at least 2 hours, or until hard.
- Store the treats in an airtight container in the refrigerator or freezer.

Nutrition:

Serving Size: 1 ball

- Calories: 100
- Carbohydrates: 15 grams
- Fat: 7 grams
- Protein: 3 grams
- Fiber: 2 grams

Tips

- For a chewier snack, add an additional 1/4 cup of oats.
- For a sweeter snack, add an additional 1 tablespoon of maple syrup.
- You may also add additional dried fruits, such raisins or blueberries, to the mixture.

10. Banana and Almond Butter Toast

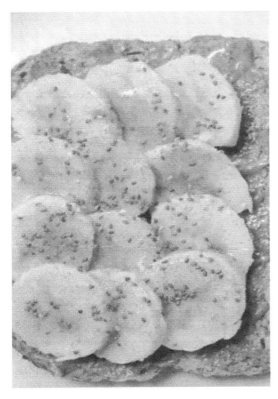

Banana and almond butter toast is a quick and simple breakfast that is both healthful and tasty. It is a fantastic source of protein, healthy fats, and fiber. The banana adds sweetness, while the almond butter delivers a rich and creamy taste. This recipe is easy to follow and may be tweaked to your desire.

Preparation Time: 5 minutes

Cooking Time: 0 minutes

Total Time: 5 minutes

Ingredients:

- 2 pieces of bread
- 1 tbsp almond butter
- 1 banana, sliced

- Optional toppings: honey, cinnamon, chia seeds, etc.

Instructions:

- Toast the bread.
- Spread the almond butter on the bread.
- Top with the banana slices.
- Sprinkle with optional toppings.
- Enjoy!

Nutrition:

Serving size: 1 slice

- Calories: 250
- Carbohydrates: 25 grams
- Fat: 15 grams
- Protein: 5 grams
- Fiber: 5 grams

Tips

- Use your preferred kind of bread.
- Mash the banana for a smoother texture.
- Add more or fewer toppings to your taste.
- Get creative with your toppings! Try adding chocolate chips, nuts, seeds, or fruit.

1. Pumpkin Spice Cheesecake Bars

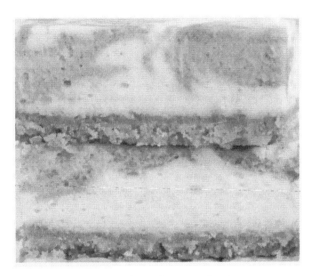

These pumpkin spice cheesecake bars are a tasty and easy-to-make treat that is great for autumn. They are prepared with a graham cracker crust, a creamy cheesecake filling, and a pumpkin spice topping. The bars are cooked till golden brown and then refrigerated until set. They are then sliced into bars and served.

Preparation Time: 20 minutes

Cooking Time: 30-35 minutes

Total Time: 50-55 minutes

Ingredients:

For the crust:

- 1 cup graham cracker crumbs
- 1/4 cup sugar
- 3 tablespoons unsalted butter, melted

For the cheesecake filling:

- 24 ounces full-fat cream cheese, softened at room temperature
- 1 cup granulated sugar
- ⅓ cup full-fat sour cream, at room temperature
- 3 big eggs, at room temperature
- 1 ½ tablespoons vanilla extract
- 1 teaspoon pumpkin pie spice

For the pumpkin spice topping:

- 1 (15 ounce) can pumpkin puree
- 1/2 cup granulated sugar
- 1 egg 1 teaspoon pumpkin pie spice

Instructions:

- Preheat the oven to 350 degrees F (175 degrees C). Grease and flour an 8x8 inch baking pan.
- In a medium bowl, mix graham cracker crumbs, sugar, and melted butter. Press into the bottom of the prepared pan.
- In a large bowl, mix cream cheese and sugar until creamy. Beat in sour cream, eggs, vanilla, and pumpkin pie spice. Pour over the crust.
- In a small bowl, mix together pumpkin puree, sugar, egg, and pumpkin pie spice. Pour over cheesecake filling.
- Bake in a preheated oven for 30-35 minutes, or until the cheesecake is set. Let cool entirely on a wire rack.
- Cut into bars and serve.

Nutrition:

Serving size: 1 bar

- Calories: 350
- Carbohydrates: 40 grams
- Fat: 15 grams
- Protein: 7 grams
- Fiber: 2 grams

Tips

- For a deeper cheesecake taste, use cream cheese that has been softened for at least 2 hours.
- To prevent the cheesecake from breaking, do not overmix the batter.
- If the cheesecake is still shaky in the middle after baking, let it cool fully before cutting.
- The cheesecake bars may be refrigerated in the refrigerator for up to 3 days.

2. Keto Brownies

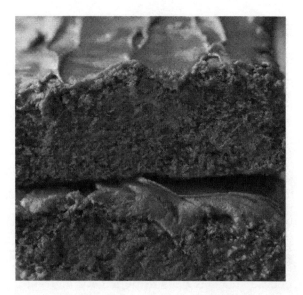

Keto brownies are a tasty and low-carb alternative to conventional brownies. They are produced using almond flour, eggs, butter, sugar replacement, and cocoa powder. Keto brownies are great for people following a keto diet or anybody searching for a healthier brownie choice.

Preparation Time: 15 minutes

Cooking Time: 30 minutes

Total Time: 45 minutes

Ingredients:

- 1 cup almond flour
- 1/2 cup cocoa powder
- 1/4 teaspoon baking powder
- 1/4 teaspoon salt
- 1/2 cup butter, melted
- 3 eggs
- 1/2 cup sugar substitute
- 1 teaspoon vanilla extract

Instructions:

- Preheat the oven to 350 degrees F (175 degrees C). Grease and flour an 8x8 inch baking pan.
- In a larger bowl, mix together the almond flour, cocoa powder, baking powder, and salt.
- In a large bowl, mix together the butter and sugar substitute until light and fluffy. Beat in the eggs one at a time, then whisk in the vanilla essence.
- Gradually add the dry ingredients to the wet components, mixing until just incorporated.
- Pour the batter into the prepared pan and bake for 30 minutes, or until a toothpick inserted into the middle comes out clean.
- Let the brownies cool fully before cutting and serving.

Nutrition:

Serving Size: 1 brownie

- Calories: 200
- Carbohydrates: 5 grams
- Fat: 15 grams
- Protein: 6 grams
- Fiber: 3 grams

Tips

- For a chewy brownie, bake for 25-30 minutes. For a fudgier brownie, bake for 30-35 minutes.
- You may use whatever sugar replacement you desire in this recipe. I prefer to use erythritol or monk fruit sweetener.
- If you don't have almond flour, you may substitute another kind of keto-friendly flour, such as coconut flour or walnut flour.
- These brownies are also wonderful topped with whipped cream, chocolate chips, or your favorite keto-friendly frosting.

3. Raspberry Sorbet

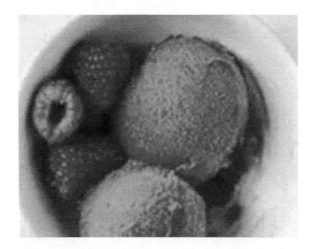

Raspberry sorbet is a tasty and refreshing frozen treat prepared with raspberries, sugar, and water. It is a terrific way to cool down on a hot day, and it is also a healthy alternative, since it is low in fat and calories.

Preparation Time: 20 minutes
Cooking Time: 10 minutes
Total Time: 30 minutes

Ingredients:

- 4 cups fresh raspberries
- 1 cup water
- 1 cup sugar
- 1 teaspoon vanilla extract

Instructions:

- Puree the raspberries in a blender or food processor until smooth.
- Strain the raspberry puree through a fine-mesh strainer to remove the seeds.

- In a medium saucepan, mix the sugar and water. Bring to a boil over medium heat, stirring frequently, until the sugar is dissolved.
- Remove the syrup from the heat and let cool slightly.
- Stir the vanilla extract into the cooled syrup.
- Combine the raspberry puree and syrup in a large bowl.
- Freeze the sorbet in an ice cream machine according to the manufacturer's directions.
- Once the sorbet is frozen, spoon it into dishes and serve.

Nutritional facts per serving:

Serving size: 1 cup

- Calories: 130
- Carbohydrates: 27 grams
- Fat: 0 grams
- Protein: 1 gram
- Fiber: 4 grams

Tips

- For a smoother sorbet, strain the raspberry puree through a fine-mesh strainer twice.
- If you don't have an ice cream machine, you may freeze the sorbet in a shallow dish. Stir it every 30 minutes to break up the ice crystals.
- You may add additional fruits to the sorbet, such as strawberries, blueberries, or blackberries.
- You may also add a dash of alcohol to the sorbet, such as raspberry liqueur or Chambord.

4. Blackberry Yogurt Popsicles

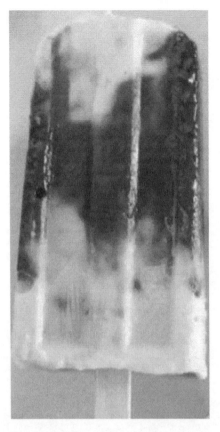

These delightful and tasty blackberry yogurt popsicles are a fantastic summer treat. They are created using basic ingredients and are easy to make. The blackberries offer a tangy flavor, while the yogurt gives them a creamy smoothness. These popsicles are a terrific way to cool down on a hot day, and they are also an excellent dose of protein and fiber.

Preparation Time: 10 minutes

Cooking Time: None

Total Time: 10 minutes

Ingredients:

- 2 cups blackberries
- 2 cups plain Greek yogurt

- 1 tablespoon lemon juice
- Popsicle sticks

Instructions:

- In a blender, purée the blackberries until smooth.
- In a medium bowl, mix together the yogurt and lemon juice.
- Fold the blackberry puree into the yogurt mixture.
- Pour the mixture into popsicle molds and insert the popsicle sticks.
- Freeze for at least 4 hours, preferably overnight.

Nutrition:

Serving size: 1 popsicle

- Calories: 100
- Carbohydrates: 17 grams
- Fat: 2 grams
- Protein: 5 grams
- Fiber: 3 grams

Tips

- For a fuller taste, use full-fat Greek yogurt.
- For a tarter taste, add additional lemon juice.
- To prepare these popsicles ahead of time, freeze them for up to 2 weeks.
- To remove the popsicles from the molds, run them under warm water for a few seconds.

5. Crumble Muffins

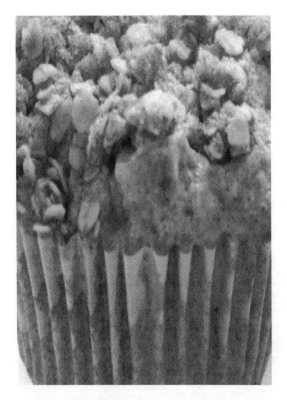

Crumble muffins are a tasty and easy-to-make delicacy that is excellent for breakfast, lunch, or a snack. They are prepared with a delicious muffin base and a crispy crumb topping. This recipe is for basic crumble muffins, but you may modify them with your favorite tastes, like chocolate chips, blueberries, or nuts.

Preparation Time: 15 minutes
Cooking Time: 20-25 minutes
Total Time: 35-40 minutes

Ingredients:

For the muffins:

- 1 1/2 cups all-purpose flour
- 1 teaspoon baking powder

- 1/2 teaspoon baking soda
- 1/4 teaspoon salt
- 1/2 cup (1 stick) unsalted butter, softened
- 1/2 cup sugar
- 1 big egg
- 1 teaspoon vanilla extract
- 1/2 cup milk

For the crumb topping:

- 1/2 cup all-purpose flour
- 1/4 cup sugar
- 1/4 teaspoon ground cinnamon
- 1/4 teaspoon salt
- 1/4 cup (1/2 stick) unsalted butter, melted

Instructions:

- Preheat the oven to 375 degrees F (190 degrees C). Grease or line a 12-cup muffin pan.
- In a large basin, mix together the flour, baking powder, baking soda, and salt.
- In a separate dish, mix together the butter and sugar until light and fluffy. Beat in the egg and vanilla extract.
- Add the dry ingredients to the wet components alternately with the milk, starting and finishing with the dry ingredients. Stir just until mixed.
- For the crumb topping, mix the flour, sugar, cinnamon, and salt in a small basin. Stir in the melted butter until crumbly.
- Divide the muffin batter equally among the prepared muffin cups. Sprinkle the crumb topping over the tops of the muffins.
- Bake for 20-25 minutes, or until a toothpick inserted into the middle of a muffin comes out clean.

- Let cool in the muffin tray for a few minutes before transferring to a wire rack to cool fully.

Nutrition:

Serving size: 1 muffin

- Calories: 250
- Carbohydrates: 35 grams
- Fat: 10 grams
- Protein: 5 grams
- Fiber: 2 grams

Tips

- For a deeper taste, use brown sugar instead of white sugar.
- Add your favorite mix-ins, such as chocolate chips, blueberries, or nuts.
- To make ahead, bake the muffins and allow them to cool fully. Store them in an airtight jar at room temperature for up to 3 days.

6. Cherry Clafoutis

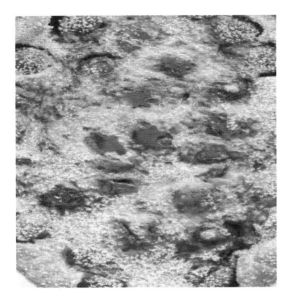

Cherry clafoutis is a popular French dessert prepared using a simple batter of eggs, milk, flour, and sugar. It is cooked in a dish with pitted cherries, and the result is a custard-like cake with a somewhat acidic taste from the cherries. Clafoutis is generally served warm or at room temperature, and it may be sprinkled with powdered sugar for an added touch of sweetness.

Preparation Time: 10 minutes
Cooking Time: 30-35 minutes
Total Time: 40-45 minutes

Ingredients:

- 2 tablespoons unsalted butter, for coating the baking dish
- 2 cups fresh delicious cherries, pitted
- 3 big eggs
- 1 cup full or 2% milk
- 1/4 cup heavy cream
- 1/2 cup granulated sugar
- 1/2 cup all-purpose flour

- 1/4 teaspoon salt
- 1/4 teaspoon vanilla extract

Instructions:

- Preheat the oven to 350 degrees F (175 degrees C). Grease a 9-inch pie plate with butter.
- Spread the cherries in the prepared pie plate.
- In a blender, mix the eggs, milk, cream, sugar, flour, salt, and vanilla extract. Blend until smooth.
- Pour the batter over the cherries.
- Bake in the preheated oven for 30-35 minutes, or until the clafoutis is golden brown and a toothpick inserted into the middle comes out clean.
- Let cool slightly before serving.

Nutrition:

This recipe produces 6 servings. Each serving comprises approximately:

- Calories: 270
- Carbohydrates: 35 grams
- Fat: 10 grams
- Protein: 8 grams
- Fiber: 2 grams

Tips

- For a deeper taste, add half & half or heavy cream instead of milk.
- If you don't have a blender, you may whisk the batter together by hand.
- To avoid the clafoutis from adhering to the edges of the baking dish, line the dish with parchment paper before adding the batter.
- Serve the clafoutis warm or at room temperature.

7. Frozen Yogurt Bark

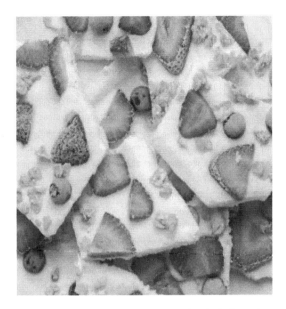

Frozen yogurt bark is a delightful and easy-to-make frozen treat. It is created with plain Greek yogurt, maple syrup, vanilla extract, and your favorite toppings. The yogurt is spread in a uniform layer on a baking sheet lined with parchment paper, and then the toppings are sprinkled on top. The bark is frozen for many hours, until it is hard, and then it is split into pieces and served.

Preparation Time: 10 minutes

Cooking Time: 0 minutes

Total Time: 10 minutes

Ingredients:

- 2 cups plain Greek yogurt
- 2 tablespoons maple syrup
- 1 teaspoon vanilla extract
- Toppings of your choosing (see below for options)

Instructions:

- Line a baking sheet with parchment paper.

- In a medium bowl, mix together the yogurt, maple syrup, and vanilla extract.

- Spread the yogurt mixture in an equal layer on the prepared baking sheet.

- Sprinkle the toppings of your choosing equally over the yogurt.

- Freeze for at least 3 hours, preferably overnight.

- Break the bark into pieces and serve.

Topping Suggestions

- Fresh berries
- Chopped nuts
- Granola Chocolate chips
- Coconut flakes
- Dried fruit

Nutrition:

Serving size: 1/4 of the bark

- Calories: 150
- Carbohydrates: 20 grams
- Fat: 5 grams
- Protein: 10 grams
- Fiber: 2 grams

Tips

- Use high-quality Greek yogurt for the greatest taste and texture.
- Don't overcrowd the baking sheet with the yogurt mixture. This will prevent the bark from freezing evenly.
- Use your favorite toppings to make a bark that is personalized to your liking.
- Store the bark in the freezer for up to 1 month.

8. Chocolate Mousse

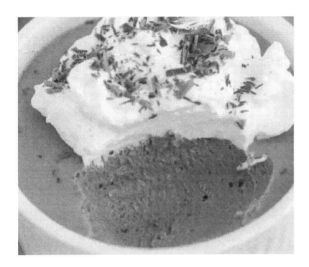

Chocolate mousse is a popular dessert that is produced with only a few basic ingredients. It is light, airy, and rich in chocolate taste. This recipe is simple to follow and provides a delectable mousse that is suitable for any occasion.

Preparation Time: 15 minutes
Cooking Time: 5 minutes
Total Time: 20 minutes

Ingredients:

- 8 ounces semisweet chocolate, chopped
- 1 cup heavy cream

- 4 big egg yolks
- ¼ cup sugar
- 4 big egg whites
- ¼ teaspoon cream of tartar

Instructions:

- Melt the chocolate in a heatproof dish put over a pot of boiling water. Stir until smooth.
- In a larger bowl, mix together the heavy cream and egg yolks. Gradually whisk in the melted chocolate until fully mixed.
- In a separate dish, whisk the egg whites and cream of tartar until soft peaks form. Gradually beat in the sugar until stiff peaks form.
- Fold the beaten egg whites into the chocolate mixture until barely incorporated.
- Pour the mousse onto individual serving plates or a big serving bowl. Chill for at least 4 hours before serving.

Nutritional facts per serving:

Serving size: 4 servings

- Calories: 300
- Carbohydrates: 25 grams
- Fat: 20 grams
- Protein: 5 grams
- Fiber: 2 grams

Tips

- For a deeper mousse, use dark chocolate instead of semisweet chocolate.
- To create individual mousse cups, line 4 ramekins with plastic wrap and fill with the mousse. Chill for at least 4 hours before serving.
- To serve, unmold mousse cups and top with whipped cream and chocolate shavings.

9. Pear and Almond Tart

Pear and almond tart is a traditional French dish that is both tasty and beautiful. The pie is constructed with a flaky pastry crust filled with a sweet and nutty frangipane filling, and topped with poached pears. It is a fantastic dessert for any occasion, and is guaranteed to amaze your guests.

Preparation Time: 30 minutes
Cooking Time: 35 minutes
Total Time: 1 hour

Ingredients:

For the pastry crust:

- 1 cup (120g) all-purpose flour
- 1/4 cup (50g) granulated sugar

- 1/4 teaspoon salt
- 1/4 cup (50g) unsalted butter, cooled and cubed
- 1 egg yolk, beaten

For the frangipane filling:

- 1/2 cup (115g) unsalted butter, softened
- 1/2 cup (100g) granulated sugar
- 1 big egg
- 1 teaspoon pure vanilla essence
- 1 cup (115g) almond flour

For the poached pears:

- 2 pears, peeled, cored, and halved
- 1 cup (240ml) water
- 1/2 cup (100g) granulated sugar
- 1/4 teaspoon ground cinnamon

Instructions:

- Preheat the oven to 375 degrees F (190 degrees C).
- To create the pastry crust, mix together the flour, sugar, and salt in a medium basin. Add the butter and use your fingers to massage it into the flour until the mixture resembles coarse crumbs. Add the egg yolk and whisk until barely blended. Form the dough into a disk, cover it in plastic wrap, and chill for at least 30 minutes.
- To prepare the frangipane filling, mix together the butter and sugar until light and fluffy. Beat in the egg and vanilla extract. Stir in the almond flour until barely incorporated.
- To poach the pears, bring the water, sugar, and cinnamon to a simmer in a small saucepan. Add the pears and poach for 15-20 minutes, or until they are soft when pricked with a fork. Remove the pears from the poaching liquid and put aside to cool.

- Roll out the pastry dough on a lightly floured board to a 12-inch circle. Transfer the dough to a 9-inch tart pan with a detachable bottom. Trim the extra dough and poke the bottom of the crust with a fork.
- Spread the frangipane filling evenly over the bottom of the crust. Top with the poached pears, cut side up.
- Bake for 30-35 minutes, or until the crust is golden brown and the filling is set. Let cool fully before serving.

Nutritional information:

Serving size: 8

- Calories: 300
- Carbohydrates: 40 grams
- Fat: 15 grams
- Protein: 5 grams
- Fiber: 5 grams

10. Berry Crumble

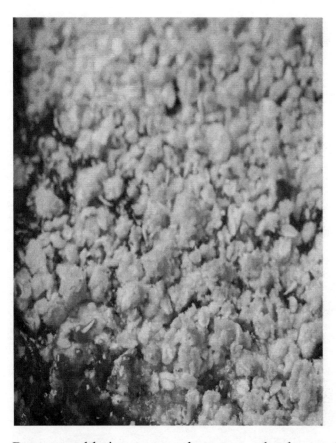

Berry crumble is a tasty and easy-to-make dessert that is excellent for any occasion. It is created with a basic fruit filling and a crispy crumble topping. This recipe is for a typical berry crumble, but you may use whatever variety of berries that you prefer.

Preparation Time: 15 minutes
Cooking Time: 30-35 minutes
Total Time: 45-50 minutes

Ingredients:

- 4 cups frozen mixed berries
- 1/2 cup sugar
- 2 tablespoons cornstarch
- 1 teaspoon lemon zest
- 1/4 teaspoon powdered cinnamon
- 1/4 teaspoon salt

- 1 cup all-purpose flour
- 1/2 cup rolled oats
- 1/4 cup brown sugar
- 1/4 cup butter, cold and cubed

Instructions:

- Preheat the oven to 375 degrees F (190 degrees C).
- In a large bowl, mix the frozen berries, sugar, cornstarch, lemon zest, cinnamon, and salt. Toss to coat.
- In a separate basin, mix the flour, oats, brown sugar, and butter. Use your fingertips or a pastry blender to massage the butter into the dry ingredients until the mixture resembles coarse crumbs.
- Pour the berry mixture into a 9x13 inch baking dish. Sprinkle the crumble topping over the berries.
- Bake in the preheated oven for 30-35 minutes, or until the topping is golden brown and the berries are bubbling.
- Serve heated or at room temperature.

Nutrition:

Serving size: 8

- Calories: 280
- Carbohydrates: 45 grams
- Fat: 10 grams
- Protein: 3 grams
- Fiber: 5 grams

Tips

- You may use any sort of berries that you prefer in this recipe.

- If you don't have frozen berries, you may substitute fresh berries. Just be careful to let them thaw before utilizing them.

- You may add additional ingredients to the crumble topping, such as almonds, seeds, or chocolate chips.

- Serve the crumble warm or at room temperature. It is also excellent served with ice cream or whipped cream.

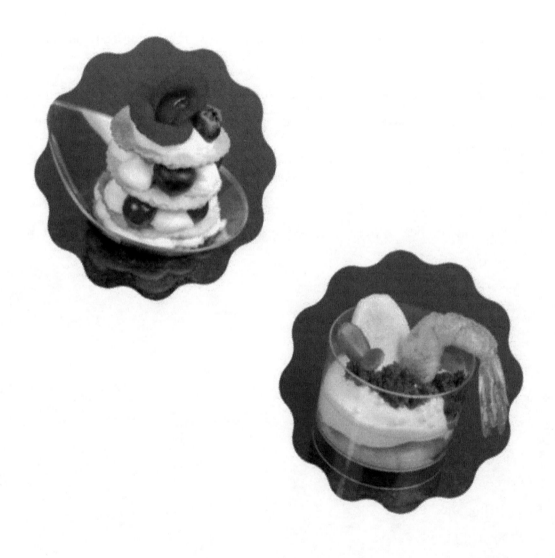

CHAPTER FIVE

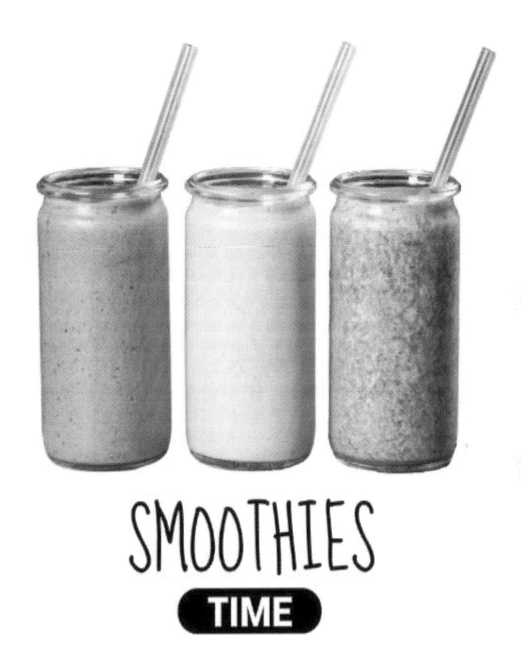

SMOOTHIES
TIME

The Ten (10) Nutritious Smoothies To Help You Boost Your Brain Power And Stay Healthy Forever

1. Beetroot Smoothie

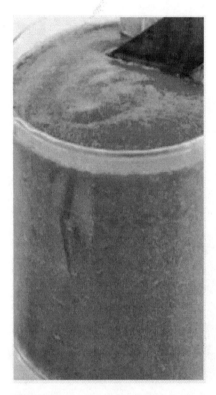

Beetroot smoothies are a tasty and healthy way to start your day. They are rich with vitamins, minerals, and antioxidants, and they may help to enhance your blood pressure, heart health, and energy levels. This dish is easy to create and only takes a few minutes to prepare.

Preparation Time: 5 minutes
Cooking Time: 0 minutes
Total Time: 5 minutes

Ingredients:

- 1 small beet, peeled and chopped

- 1 apple, cored and cut
- 1 banana, sliced
- 1 cup of frozen berries
- 1/2 cup of milk or yogurt
- 1/4 cup of water
- Ice cubes, to taste

Instructions:

- Add all of the ingredients to a blender and mix until smooth.
- Serve immediately or keep in an airtight jar in the refrigerator for up to 24 hours.

Nutrition:

Serve Size: 1 serve

- Calories: 250
- Carbohydrates: 40 grams
- Fat: 5 grams
- Protein: 10 grams
- Fiber: 5 grams

Tips

- If you don't have a high-powered blender, you may roast the beet before blending to make it simpler to purée.
- You may add additional ingredients to the smoothie, such as spinach, ginger, or chia seeds.
- Enjoy your smoothie now or save it in the refrigerator for later.

2. Peanut Butter Banana Smoothie

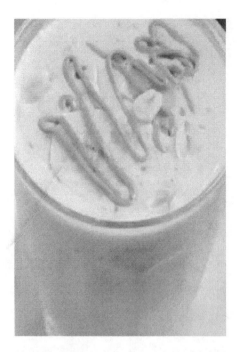

Peanut butter banana smoothies are a wonderful and healthful way to start your day. They are rich with protein, fiber, and healthy fats, and they are a fantastic source of potassium and vitamin C. This dish is fast and simple to create, and it only takes a few ingredients.

Preparation Time: 5 minutes

Cooking Time: 0 minutes

Total Time: 5 minutes

Ingredients:

- 1 frozen banana, cut
- 1/2 cup milk
- 2 tbsp peanut butter
- 1 teaspoon vanilla extract
- 1/4 teaspoon ground cinnamon
- Ice cubes, optional

Instructions:

- Place all of the ingredients in a blender and mix until smooth.
- If the smoothie is too thick, add extra milk or ice cubes.
- Pour and enjoy!

Nutritional information:

Serving size: 1 smoothie

- Calories: 350
- Carbohydrates: 40 grams
- Fat: 15 grams
- Protein: 10 grams
- Fiber: 5 grams

Tips

- For a thicker smoothie, use less milk or add more ice cubes.
- For a sweeter smoothie, add extra banana or a sweetener of your choosing.
- For a more protein-rich smoothie, add a scoop of protein powder.
- You may also add additional components to your smoothie, such as berries, oats, or chia seeds.

3. Spinach Smoothie

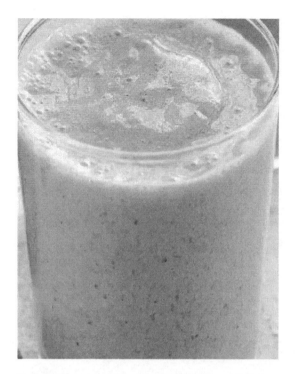

Spinach smoothies are a terrific way to get your daily dosage of veggies in a tasty and refreshing manner. They are also an excellent source of protein, fiber, and other nutrients. This recipe is for a simple spinach smoothie that you can modify with your favorite fruits and add-ins.

Preparation Time: 5 minutes

Cooking Time: 0 minutes

Total Time: 5 minutes

Ingredients:

- 1 cup baby spinach
- 1/2 cup frozen banana, chopped
- 1/2 cup milk (any sort)
- 1/4 cup Greek yogurt (any flavor)
- 1 tablespoon honey (optional)

Instructions:

- Add all ingredients to a blender and mix until smooth.
- Adjust sweetness with honey, if desired.
- Serve immediately.

Nutrition (per serving):

Serving size: 1 cup

- Calories: 180
- Carbohydrates: 25 grams
- Fat: 5 grams
- Protein: 10 grams
- Fiber: 5 grams

Tips

- Use frozen spinach for a richer smoothie.
- Add more fruits, such as berries, mango, or pineapple, for a sweeter smoothie.
- Add a scoop of protein powder for a more satisfying smoothie.
- Adjust the quantity of honey to taste.

4. Strawberry Banana Smoothie

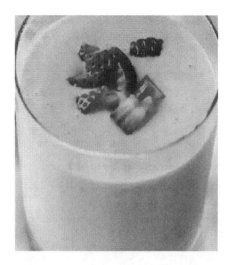

Strawberry banana smoothies are a tasty and nutritious way to start your day. They are rich with vitamins, minerals, and antioxidants, and they are a fantastic source of fiber. This dish is fast and easy to create, and it only takes a few basic ingredients.

Preparation Time: 5 minutes
Cooking Time: 0 minutes
Total Time: 5 minutes

Ingredients:

- 2 cups frozen strawberries
- 1 banana, frozen
- 1 cup milk (any variety)
- 1/2 cup yogurt (any kind)
- Optional: 1 teaspoon vanilla extract

Instructions:

- Combine all items in a blender.

- Blend until smooth.
- Enjoy!

Nutritional information:

Serving size: 1 smoothie

- Calories: 250
- Carbohydrates: 40 grams
- Fat: 5 grams
- Protein: 8 grams
- Fiber: 5 grams

Tips

- For a thicker smoothie, add extra frozen strawberries or ice.
- For a thinner smoothie, add extra milk or yogurt.
- Add additional fruits or vegetables, such as blueberries, raspberries, spinach, or kale.
- Add a sweetener, such as honey, maple syrup, or agave nectar.
- Top with granola, nuts, or seeds.

5. Mango Pineapple Smoothie

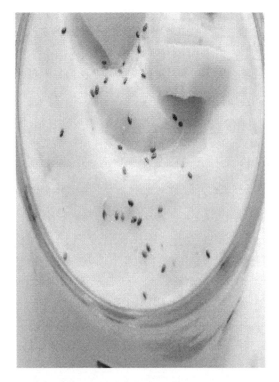

This delightful smoothie is composed with frozen mango, pineapple, yogurt, and honey. It's a tasty and healthful way to start your day, or enjoy as a snack.

Preparation Time: 5 minutes

Cooking Time: 0 minutes

Total Time: 5 minutes

Ingredients:

- 1 cup frozen mango chunks
- 1 cup frozen pineapple chunks
- 1/2 cup plain yogurt
- 1 tablespoon honey
- Ice cubes, to taste

Instructions:

- Combine all items in a blender.
- Blend until smooth and creamy.
- Serve immediately.

Nutritional information:

Serving size: 1 cup

- Calories: 250
- Carbohydrates: 45 grams
- Fat: 5 grams
- Protein: 5 grams
- Fiber: 5 grams

Tips

- You may add fresh mango and pineapple if you want, but frozen fruits will make the smoothie thicker and creamier.
- If you prefer a sweeter smoothie, add additional honey to taste.
- You may also add additional fruits to the smoothie, such as banana, strawberry, or peach.

6. Acai Berry Smoothie

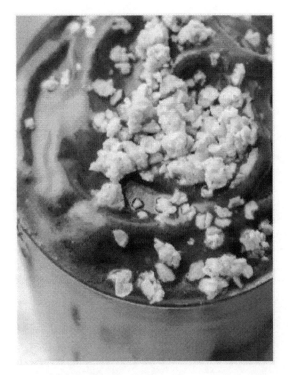

Acai berry smoothies are a tasty and nutritious way to start your day. They are filled with antioxidants and other minerals, and they are a fantastic source of fiber. This dish is simple to create and may be tweaked to your desire.

Preparation Time: 5 minutes
Cooking Time: 0 minutes
Total Time: 5 minutes

Ingredients:

- 1 cup frozen acai berries
- 1 cup frozen mixed berries (such as blueberries, raspberries, and strawberries)
- 1 banana, sliced
- 1 cup almond milk or other plant milk
- 1 tablespoon honey or maple syrup (optional).

Instructions:

- Add all of the ingredients to a blender.
- Blend until smooth.
- Pour into a glass and enjoy!

Nutritional information:

Serving size: 1 smoothie

- Calories: 300
- Carbohydrates: 50 grams
- Fat: 10 grams
- Protein: 5 grams
- Fiber: 10 grams

Tips

- You may use fresh or frozen acai berries.
- If you don't have almond milk, you may substitute any other plant milk, such as soy milk, oat milk, or rice milk.
- You may alter the sweetness of the smoothie to your desire by adding more or less honey or maple syrup.
- You may also add additional ingredients to the smoothie, such as chia seeds, protein powder, or granola.

7. Banana Walnut Smoothie

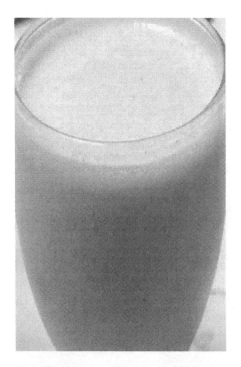

This banana walnut smoothie is a delightful and healthful breakfast or snack choice. It is created using basic ingredients that are filled with nutrients. The bananas supply potassium and fiber, the walnuts provide heart-healthy fats, and the milk provides protein. This smoothie is simple to prepare and may be tweaked to your desire.

Preparation Time: 5 minutes
Cooking Time: 0 minutes
Total Time: 5 minutes

Ingredients:

- 1 frozen banana
- 1 cup milk of choice (almond milk, soy milk, or dairy milk)
- ⅓ cup walnuts
- ¼ teaspoon cinnamon (optional)

Instructions:

- Add all items to a blender.
- Blend on high speed until smooth.
- Pour into a glass and enjoy!

Nutritional information:

Serving size: 1 smoothie

- Calories: 250
- Carbohydrates: 35 grams
- Fat: 10 grams
- Protein: 8 grams
- Fiber: 5 grams

Tips

- For a sweeter smoothie, add a spoonful of honey or maple syrup.
- For a thicker smoothie, add a handful of ice cubes.
- You may also add additional ingredients to this smoothie, such as berries, spinach, or protein powder.

8. Green Smoothie

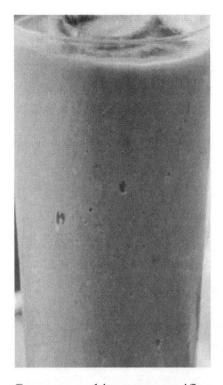

Green smoothies are a terrific way to obtain your daily dosage of fruits, veggies, and minerals. They are simple to prepare and may be tailored to your own liking. This recipe for a green smoothie is easy and tasty. It is created with spinach, banana, mango, and almond milk. The smoothie is rich with vitamins, minerals, and antioxidants. It is a terrific way to start your day or as a nutritious snack.

Preparation Time: 5 minutes

Cooking Time: 0 minutes

Total Time: 5 minutes

Ingredients:

- 1 cup spinach
- 1 banana
- 1/2 cup mango, frozen or fresh

- 1/2 cup almond milk
- 1/4 teaspoon ground cinnamon (optional)

Instructions:

- Place all ingredients in a blender and mix until smooth.
- Pour into a glass and enjoy!

Nutritions:

Serve Size: 1 serve

- Calories: 250
- Carbohydrates: 40 grams
- Fat: 10 grams
- Protein: 5 grams
- Fiber: 5 grams

Tips

- Use frozen mango for a thicker smoothie.
- Add extra fruits or vegetables, such as berries, kale, or avocado.
- Use your preferred milk, such as dairy milk, soy milk, or almond milk.
- Adjust the quantity of cinnamon to taste.

9. Ginger Turmeric Smoothie

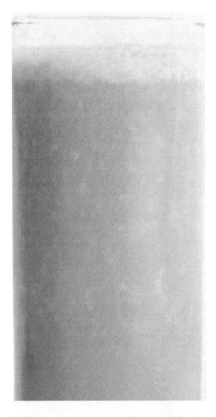

Ginger Turmeric Smoothie is a tasty and healthy way to start your day. It is filled with antioxidants and anti-inflammatory components, which may help strengthen your immune system, improve your digestion, and decrease inflammation. This smoothie is also vegan and gluten-free, making it a perfect alternative for anyone with dietary limitations.

Preparation Time: 5 minutes

Cooking Time: 0 minutes

Total Time: 5 minutes

Ingredients:

- 1 huge ripe banana, peeled and sliced
- 1 cup frozen or fresh pineapple
- 1/2 tablespoon fresh ginger, peeled and grated

- 1/4 teaspoon ground turmeric
- 1/2 cup unsweetened almond milk
- 1 tablespoon lemon juice

Instructions:

- Combine all ingredients in a blender and mix until smooth.
- Pour into a glass and enjoy!

Nutrition:

Serve size: 1 serve

- Calories: 250
- Carbohydrates: 40 grams
- Fat: 5 grams
- Protein: 5 grams
- Fiber: 5 grams

Tips

- For a sweeter smoothie, add additional bananas.
- For a more tart smoothie, add extra lemon juice.
- For a thicker smoothie, use less almond milk.
- You may also add additional ingredients to this smoothie, such as spinach, avocado, or yogurt.

10. Blueberry Avocado Smoothie

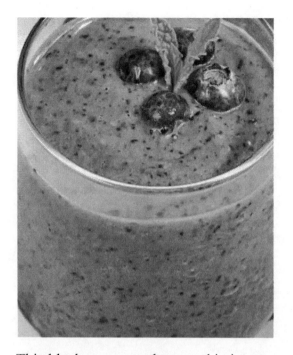

This blueberry avocado smoothie is a tasty and healthful way to start your day. It is created with a blend of fresh or frozen blueberries, ripe avocado, almond milk, and banana. The avocado offers a creamy texture and healthful fats, while the blueberries and banana bring sweetness and antioxidants. This smoothie is also a wonderful source of protein and fiber.

Preparation Time: 5 minutes
Cooking Time: 0 minutes
Total Time: 5 minutes

Ingredients:

- 1 cup frozen blueberries
- 1/2 ripe avocado, peeled and pitted
- 1 banana, peeled
- 1 cup almond milk
- Optional: 1 tablespoon chia seeds, hemp seeds, or ground flaxseed

Instructions:

- Place all ingredients in a blender and mix until smooth.
- Enjoy instantly.

Nutritional information:

Serving size: 1 cup

- Calories: 350
- Carbohydrates: 35 grams
- Fat: 15 grams
- Protein: 8 grams
- Fiber: 10 grams

Tips

- For a thicker smoothie, add a handful of ice.
- For a thinner smoothie, add additional almond milk.
- You may also add different fruits, such as strawberries, raspberries, or mango.
- If you prefer a sweeter smoothie, add a teaspoon of honey or maple syrup.

Ten (10) Different Cognitive Exercises To Help You Improve Your Brain Health

Here are 10 different activities that may help you enhance your cognitive health:

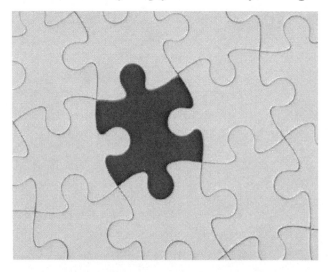

1. Jigsaw puzzles. Jigsaw puzzles are a terrific method to strengthen your visual-spatial abilities, problem-solving skills, and memory.

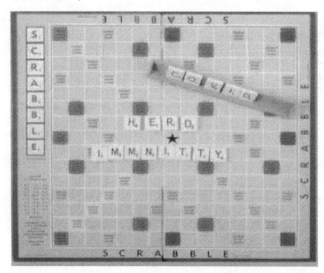

2. Word games. Word games like crossword puzzles, Scrabble, and Boggle may help increase your vocabulary, word memory, and problem-solving abilities.

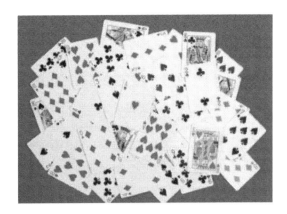

3. Card games. Card games like bridge, poker, and solitaire may help enhance your memory, concentration, and problem-solving abilities.

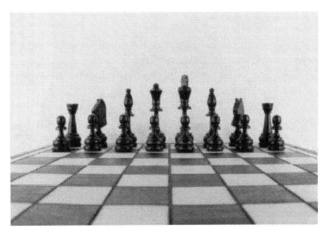

4. Sudoku. Sudoku is a logic puzzle that may enhance your problem-solving abilities, focus, and short-term memory.

5. Chess. Chess is a strategic board game that may enhance your problem-solving abilities, critical thinking, and long-term memory.

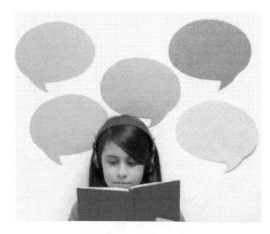

6. Learning a new language. Learning a new language may assist increase your memory, concentration, and cognitive flexibility.

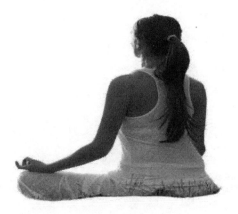

7. Meditation. Meditation may enhance your attention, concentration, and emotional management.

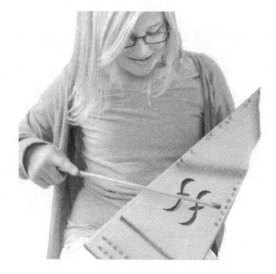

8. Playing an instrument. Playing an instrument may enhance your hand-eye coordination, memory, and problem-solving abilities.

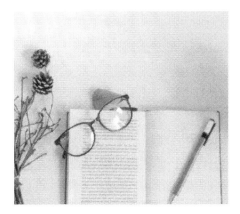

9. Reading. Reading may assist in increasing your vocabulary, comprehension, and critical thinking abilities.

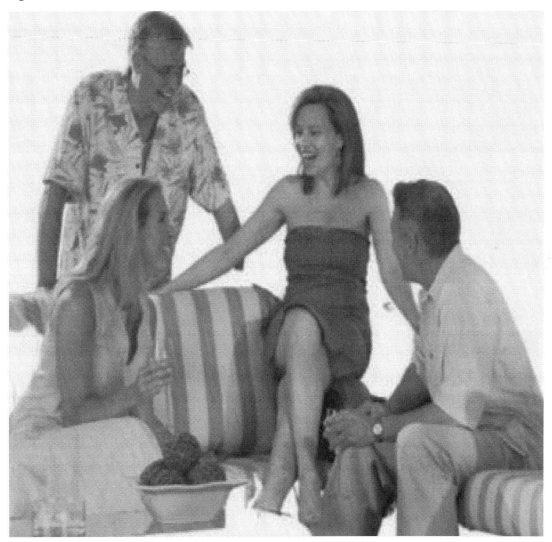

10. Socializing. Socializing may assist increase your memory, concentration, and cognitive flexibility.

These are just a few examples of cognitive exercises that you may undertake to boost your brain health. There are many different workouts available, so select those that you love and that challenge you. The more you do, the better your cognitive health will be.

Here are some other strategies for enhancing your cognitive health:

- Get adequate sleep.
- Eat a nutritious diet.
- Exercise frequently.
- Manage stress.
- Stay socially engaged.
- Challenge yourself cognitively.

By following these guidelines, you may help maintain your brain healthy and bright for years to come.

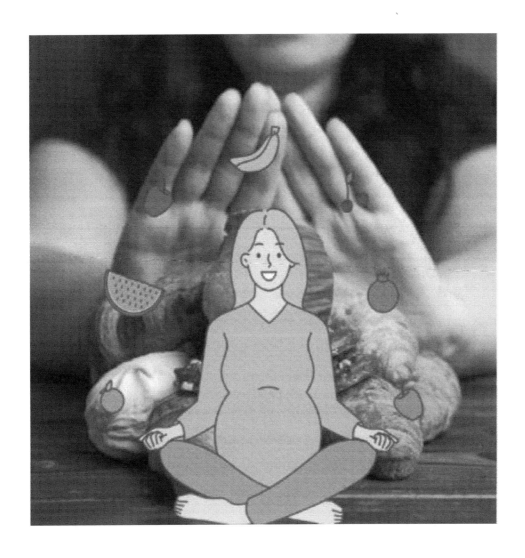

How To Make The MIND Diet Easy to Follow

The MIND diet is not difficult to follow, but it does take some forethought. Here are some ways to make it easier:

1. Start by making tiny modifications. Don't attempt to alter your whole diet overnight. Start by adding one or two MIND-approved items to your meals each day.

2. Make it a family affair. If everyone in your home is on board with the MIND diet, it will be much simpler to adhere to it. Get your kids involved in meal planning and preparing, and make sure there are always plenty of MIND-approved snacks available.

3. Find recipes that you adore. There are numerous tasty MIND-approved dishes accessible online and in cookbooks. Find a handful that you truly appreciate, and make them a regular part of your meal rotation.

4. Don't be scared to improvise. If you don't have all the ingredients for a MIND-approved dish, don't be scared to adapt. There are many different methods to create nutritious, brain-friendly meals.

5. Don't beat yourself up if you slip up. Everyone makes errors. If you have a day when you don't keep to the MIND diet, don't beat yourself up. Just get back on track the following day.

The MIND diet is a long-term commitment, but it's worth it for your brain health. By following these recommendations, you may make it simpler to adhere to the MIND diet and get the advantages for years to come.

Here are some more recommendations to make the MIND diet simple to follow:

1. Shop for MIND-approved foods. When you're at the grocery store, be sure to load up on MIND-approved foods like leafy green veggies, berries, nuts, whole grains, salmon, and legumes.

2. Cook at home more frequently. This will offer you greater control over the components in your meals.

3. Read food labels carefully. Look for foods that are low in saturated fat, trans fat, and added sugar.

4. Be aware of your portion amounts. It's easy to overeat, so be cautious of how much food you're placing on your plate.

5. Make incremental modifications. Don't attempt to modify your whole diet overnight. Start by making tiny modifications, then gradually increase your consumption of MIND-approved meals.

Following the MIND diet is a terrific approach to boost your brain health and lower your risk of Alzheimer's disease. By following these recommendations, you may make it simpler to adhere to the MIND diet and get the advantages for years to come.

How To Adapt The MIND Diet For Your Needs

There are a few methods to adjust the MIND diet for your unique requirements. Here are some tips:

1. Consider your dietary constraints. If you have any dietary constraints, such as allergies or intolerances, you may still follow the MIND diet. There are several substitutions that you may use to meet your requirements. For example, if you are allergic to nuts, you may replace seeds or legumes.

2. Take your lifestyle into consideration. If you are busy or don't love cooking, you may still follow the MIND diet. There are several simple and practical ways to add MIND-approved foods into your diet. For example, you may purchase pre-cut veggies, frozen berries, or canned beans.

3. Make incremental modifications. If you are accustomed to consuming a lot of processed foods, it may be tough to make a rapid adjustment to the MIND diet. Instead, make modest modifications over time. For example, start by adding one or two MIND-approved meals to your diet each week.

How To Stay Motivated On The MIND Diet

If you're thinking about starting the MIND diet, it's crucial to keep motivated. Here are a few tips:

1. Set reasonable objectives. Don't attempt to modify your whole diet overnight. Start by making little adjustments, such as adding extra leafy greens to your meals or changing out sugary snacks for fruits.

2. Find a support system. Having friends or family members who are also on the MIND diet might help you keep on track. You may exchange recipes, advice, and encourage one other through the trials.

3. Make it simple. Stock your kitchen with MIND-approved meals so that you don't have to make a lot of complex selections when you're hungry. Keep fruits, veggies, healthy grains, and lean protein on hand.

4. Don't be scared to indulge. The MIND diet doesn't mean you have to give up all of your favorite foods. Just be sure to consume in moderation.

5. Track your progress. Keeping track of your progress might help you remain motivated. You may use a food diary or an app to document what you eat and how you feel.

CONCLUSION

The Mind Diet Cookbook is a complete resource for anybody wishing to enhance their mental health via nutrition. The Mind Diet is based on the premise that particular meals may aid to boost brain function and lower the risk of cognitive decline.

The diet emphasizes complete, unprocessed foods that are rich in nutrients that are vital for brain function. These include fruits, vegetables, nutritious grains, healthy fats, and lean protein.

If you are wanting to enhance your mental health via eating, the Mind Diet Cookbook is a terrific place to start. The book is full of information and recipes that will enable you to make healthy decisions that will improve your brain.

There Is No Further Information!

Thank you for ordering this book **"Mind Diet Cookbook For Seniors"** and I hope that you like it.

If you have an experience with the book that you would want to share with me, I would highly appreciate it!

Please take a minute to write me a "FAVORABLE REVIEW" on the site on which you bought the book or any other online review community. By providing me the chance to gather feedback from you, you will assist to make this book better for future readers and help to broaden its reach.

When you finish your review, please add any comments on how I may improve this book. I am continuously working to make it the best that it can be for my readers.

To show my appreciation, I am offering a complimentary email consultation to answer any questions you may have about this book. Maybe you're confused on a certain concept or require help understanding it better - I'm Here To Help.

To take advantage of this offer, just drop me an email at jhendersonanne@gmail.com with the title "Book Consultation" and a brief description of whatever issue you need help with. I will do my best to get back to you within 24 hours with a useful response.

Don't forget to post a review on this book.

Thank You For Making This Purchase And I Look Forward To Your Email.

20 Pages Of Meal Planner

&

10 Pages Of Shopping List

Journal

FOOD JOURNAL

Breakfast	Servings	Calories
	Subtotal	

Snack		
	Subtotal	

Lunch		
	Subtotal	

Snack		
	Subtotal	

Dinner		
	Subtotal	

Snack		
	Subtotal	

Total Calories From Food [   ]

FITNESS ACTIVITY JOURNAL

	Duration	Calories

Total Calories From Fitness [   ]

NOTES

FOOD JOURNAL

Breakfast	Servings	Calories
	Subtotal	

Snack		
	Subtotal	

Lunch		
	Subtotal	

Snack		
	Subtotal	

Dinner		
	Subtotal	

Snack		
	Subtotal	

Total Calories From Food	

FITNESS ACTIVITY JOURNAL

	Duration	Calories
Total Calories From Fitness		

NOTES

FOOD JOURNAL

Breakfast	Servings	Calories	
		Subtotal	

Snack			
		Subtotal	

Lunch			
		Subtotal	

Snack			
		Subtotal	

Dinner			
		Subtotal	

Snack			
		Subtotal	

Total Calories From Food

FITNESS ACTIVITY JOURNAL

	Duration	Calories

Total Calories From Fitness

NOTES

FOOD JOURNAL

Breakfast	Servings	Calories
	Subtotal	

Snack		
	Subtotal	

Lunch		
	Subtotal	

Snack		
	Subtotal	

Dinner		
	Subtotal	

Snack		
	Subtotal	

Total Calories From Food	

FITNESS ACTIVITY JOURNAL

	Duration	Calories
Total Calories From Fitness		

NOTES

FOOD JOURNAL

Breakfast	Servings	Calories
	Subtotal	

Snack	Servings	Calories
	Subtotal	

Lunch	Servings	Calories
	Subtotal	

Snack	Servings	Calories
	Subtotal	

Dinner	Servings	Calories
	Subtotal	

Snack	Servings	Calories
	Subtotal	

Total Calories From Food

FITNESS ACTIVITY JOURNAL

	Duration	Calories

Total Calories From Fitness

NOTES

FOOD JOURNAL

Breakfast	Servings	Calories
		Subtotal

Snack		
		Subtotal

Lunch		
		Subtotal

Snack		
		Subtotal

Dinner		
		Subtotal

Snack		
		Subtotal

Total Calories From Food

FITNESS ACTIVITY JOURNAL

	Duration	Calories

Total Calories From Fitness

NOTES

FOOD JOURNAL

Breakfast	Servings	Calories
	Subtotal	

Snack		
	Subtotal	

Lunch		
	Subtotal	

Snack		
	Subtotal	

Dinner		
	Subtotal	

Snack		
	Subtotal	

Total Calories From Food

FITNESS ACTIVITY JOURNAL

	Duration	Calories

Total Calories From Fitness

NOTES

FOOD JOURNAL

Breakfast	Servings	Calories
	Subtotal	

Snack		
	Subtotal	

Lunch		
	Subtotal	

Snack		
	Subtotal	

Dinner		
	Subtotal	

Snack		
	Subtotal	

Total Calories From Food

FITNESS ACTIVITY JOURNAL

	Duration	Calories

Total Calories From Fitness

NOTES

FOOD JOURNAL

Breakfast	Servings	Calories
	Subtotal	

Snack		
	Subtotal	

Lunch		
	Subtotal	

Snack		
	Subtotal	

Dinner		
	Subtotal	

Snack		
	Subtotal	

Total Calories From Food

FITNESS ACTIVITY JOURNAL

	Duration	Calories

Total Calories From Fitness

NOTES

FOOD JOURNAL

Breakfast	Servings	Calories	
		Subtotal	

Snack			
		Subtotal	

Lunch			
		Subtotal	

Snack			
		Subtotal	

Dinner			
		Subtotal	

Snack			
		Subtotal	

Total Calories From Food

FITNESS ACTIVITY JOURNAL

	Duration	Calories

Total Calories From Fitness

NOTES

FOOD JOURNAL

Breakfast	Servings	Calories
	Subtotal	

Snack		
	Subtotal	

Lunch		
	Subtotal	

Snack		
	Subtotal	

Dinner		
	Subtotal	

Snack		
	Subtotal	

Total Calories From Food

FITNESS ACTIVITY JOURNAL

	Duration	Calories
Total Calories From Fitness		

NOTES

FOOD JOURNAL

Breakfast		Servings	Calories
		Subtotal	

Snack			
		Subtotal	

Lunch			
		Subtotal	

Snack			
		Subtotal	

Dinner			
		Subtotal	

Snack			
		Subtotal	

Total Calories From Food

FITNESS ACTIVITY JOURNAL

	Duration	Calories

Total Calories From Fitness

NOTES

FOOD JOURNAL

Breakfast	Servings	Calories
	Subtotal	

Snack		
	Subtotal	

Lunch		
	Subtotal	

Snack		
	Subtotal	

Dinner		
	Subtotal	

Snack		
	Subtotal	

Total Calories From Food

FITNESS ACTIVITY JOURNAL

	Duration	Calories

Total Calories From Fitness

NOTES

FOOD JOURNAL

Breakfast		Servings	Calories	
		Subtotal		

Snack				
		Subtotal		

Lunch				
		Subtotal		

Snack				
		Subtotal		

Dinner				
		Subtotal		

Snack				
		Subtotal		

Total Calories From Food

FITNESS ACTIVITY JOURNAL

	Duration	Calories

Total Calories From Fitness

NOTES

FOOD JOURNAL

Breakfast	Servings	Calories	
		Subtotal	

Snack			
		Subtotal	

Lunch			
		Subtotal	

Snack			
		Subtotal	

Dinner			
		Subtotal	

Snack			
		Subtotal	

Total Calories From Food [ ]

FITNESS ACTIVITY JOURNAL

	Duration	Calories

Total Calories From Fitness [ ]

NOTES

FOOD JOURNAL

Breakfast	Servings	Calories	
		Subtotal	

Snack			
		Subtotal	

Lunch			
		Subtotal	

Snack			
		Subtotal	

Dinner			
		Subtotal	

Snack			
		Subtotal	
		Total Calories From Food	

FITNESS ACTIVITY JOURNAL

	Duration	Calories
Total Calories From Fitness		

NOTES

FOOD JOURNAL

Breakfast	Servings	Calories	
		Subtotal	

Snack			
		Subtotal	

Lunch			
		Subtotal	

Snack			
		Subtotal	

Dinner			
		Subtotal	

Snack			
		Subtotal	

Total Calories From Food [ ]

FITNESS ACTIVITY JOURNAL

	Duration	Calories

Total Calories From Fitness [ ]

NOTES

FOOD JOURNAL

Breakfast	Servings	Calories
	Subtotal	

Snack		
	Subtotal	

Lunch		
	Subtotal	

Snack		
	Subtotal	

Dinner		
	Subtotal	

Snack		
	Subtotal	

Total Calories From Food [ ]

FITNESS ACTIVITY JOURNAL

	Duration	Calories

Total Calories From Fitness [ ]

NOTES

FOOD JOURNAL

Breakfast	Servings	Calories
	Subtotal	

Snack		
	Subtotal	

Lunch		
	Subtotal	

Snack		
	Subtotal	

Dinner		
	Subtotal	

Snack		
	Subtotal	

Total Calories From Food

FITNESS ACTIVITY JOURNAL

	Duration	Calories

Total Calories From Fitness

NOTES

FOOD JOURNAL

Breakfast	Servings	Calories
	Subtotal	

Snack		
	Subtotal	

Lunch		
	Subtotal	

Snack		
	Subtotal	

Dinner		
	Subtotal	

Snack		
	Subtotal	

Total Calories From Food

FITNESS ACTIVITY JOURNAL

	Duration	Calories

Total Calories From Fitness

NOTES

Shopping List

Vegetables

Fruits

Protein

Dairy

Snacks

Dry Goods

Shopping List

Vegetables

Fruits

Protein

Dairy

Snacks

Dry Goods

Shopping List

Vegetables

Fruits

Protein

Dairy

Snacks

Dry Goods

Shopping List

Vegetables

Fruits

Protein

Dairy

Snacks

Dry Goods

Shopping List

Vegetables

Fruits

Protein

Dairy

Snacks

Dry Goods

Shopping List

Vegetables

Fruits

Protein

Dairy

Snacks

Dry Goods

Shopping List

Vegetables

Fruits

Protein

Dairy

Snacks

Dry Goods

Shopping List

Vegetables

Fruits

Protein

Dairy

Snacks

Dry Goods

Shopping List

Vegetables

Fruits

Protein

Dairy

Snacks

Dry Goods

Shopping List

Vegetables

Fruits

Protein

Dairy

Snacks

Dry Goods

Made in the USA
Monee, IL
10 April 2024

56724180R00120